Praise for *A Woman's Guide to Saving Her Own Life*

Mellanie True Hills has written an engaging, compelling book that will save lives. Her story could be any woman's story, so it is important that we all know what to do to protect ourselves. As a journalist, I read many health stories and hear many personal tales of survival, but none have been so helpful and "from the heart" as Mellanie's.

—Lorri Allen, News Director, FamilyNet

A Woman's Guide to Saving Her Own Life is both informative and inspirational. Every woman should do herself a favor and read this book to learn more about living healthfully.

—Jess Brittain, Host, The Women's Room, WGLS Radio

You can't help but think that "this could've been me" when reading Mellanie's story—you see resemblances to your own life. Being in high-tech, like Mellanie, I resonate with her experience. We are "over-achievers at work," never saying NO, being "Super Mom" at home, and multitasking so that there is never any idle time. Sometimes, the stress of all these things motivates us, but can kill us.

Mellanie unselfishly took her frightening experience and provided us a roadmap to detect the early warning signs of heart problems. Not only does she provide the medical research in a "user-friendly" format but she also provides a plan on how to save your life. She coaches you on how to change from destructive and stressful behavior to a calmer and more peaceful lifestyle. This is a book that I will refer to time and time again. Thank goodness for this book and the tools and skills to adopt better health, personal growth, and inner peace in a hurried world.

—Debra Brown, United Nations Department of Peacekeeping Operations, in Liberia

With more women dying from heart disease than breast cancer, it's gratifying to see someone making a strong and intelligent effort to warn us about "The Silent Killer." Mellanie True Hills is a delight to interview and explains the deadly challenge in everyday language.

—Jim Cox, News Director, KEZK, St. Louis, MO

Mellanie turned her personal story into a road map to give women the knowledge to lead healthier lives.

—Sharon Frey, Subway Franchisee Advertising Fund, Austin Market, Board Chair

A great mix of personal stories and facts and a terrific sense of humor!

—Gayle Golladay

The book is filled with nuts and bolts common sense ideas to help women take charge of their own health! A must for every woman concerned about her well-being!

—Bob Gourley, Issues Today, http://issuestodayradio.com

Throughout, the book is conversational, speaks right to the reader, and is so easy to understand. I learned that high blood pressure and cold weather don't mix! It's a job well done...the layout, the look, and the amazing facts.

—Diane Graden, Always Right/Customer Service Solutions, www.alwaysright.biz

A Woman's Guide to Saving Her Own Life was hard to put down—every time I put it down, it called me back. I'm reading it for a second time and enjoying it just as much.

—Joyce Hills

Mellanie's own story and the facts that she presents scared me into recognizing that today's bad habits can be tomorrow's life-threatening health issues. Fortunately, she provides us with a robust but easily understood explanation of heart disease and its causes, as well as a logical plan for taking control of our heart health. Written in layperson's terms, the book provides more than just explanations—it provides a wealth of tools such as a risk factors worksheet, goal setting tools, and detailed information on how to eat healthy without sacrificing taste. In short, A Woman's Guide to Saving Her Own Life is a must read for any woman intent on avoiding the pitfalls of heart disease, or for anyone who wants to make a positive impact on their health.

—Karen Hiser, http://www.HealthyTravelNetwork.com

This book had better grab the attention of Type A women and their families who think they are invincible! Type A women who think they are immune to heart disease because it does not run in their families had better rethink that fallacy too. Mellanie True Hills has delivered the women's "heart" book that is already saving lives. Her own story is fascinating, and yes I knew Mellanie before and after her episode. This book truly reveals God's purpose for Mellanie's life. Her intelligence, knowledge, underlying competency, and writing skill evoke the passion and dedication that will be the hallmark for the rest of her prolific life. It is with pride and joy for my Leadership Texas 2003 sister that I recommend this book. Mellanie is doing for women's heart disease what other women have done for breast cancer—getting the REAL facts out ma'am!

—Susan Macaulay, Richardson, Texas

I passed this book along to my mother, who has read and GREATLY appreciates Mellanie's perseverance to document her story. My mother very recently experienced what Mellanie did, had a stent put in place, and is grateful to know she's not alone in her journey.

—Lisa McNew, CEO, Alliance of Technology and Women International

A Woman's Guide to Saving Her Own Life can do precisely what the title says. Mellanie's story is so many women's story. The book is so useful because it relates to all of us but goes one step further. The reality of women's heart issues is paramount to increasing awareness and having an impact on women becoming their own health advocates. It provides the steps necessary to make the changes.

Clients contact me when they need to make a change. Initially the intensity for making change is high and it fuels their motivation. Client motivation often decreases over the course of time. Mellanie's book is a great reminder and a way to keep that motivation.

All women can identify with Mellanie's story. Her experience can assist them with one of the biggest challenges we face—taking care of ourselves in order to take care of others. By providing them with the necessary knowledge and a plan, this book will help women save their own lives.

—Nina Rowan, CEO, Rowan Health Concepts, www.rowanhealth.com

A Woman's Guide to Saving Her Own Life is informative and helpful and written so that anyone might easily understand and then follow the advice. As the author has been through this jungle and back, she gently guides you through what could be pitfalls for the uninitiated. I like her writing style—it's like having an intimate conversation with a good friend.

—Claudia Snow, Owner, Snow Construction Company

Our children, friends, family and colleagues depend on us. With health problems in my family history, I hadn't owned finding a solution. Thanks for showing us how we can be there in the future. If you are a woman, and you want to be around and active for the rest of your life, you must read this book. There is no telling how many women will make the choices now to be around later.

—Linda Byars Swindling, JD, Author of *The Consultant's Legal Guide* and National Director of the National Speakers Association

A Woman's Guide to Saving Her Own Life

The HEART Program
for Health and Longevity

Mellanie True Hills
The Health & Productivity Revitalizer®

Healthy Ideas Press • Greenwood, Texas

A Woman's Guide to Saving Her Own Life
The HEART Program for Health and Longevity

by Mellanie True Hills
The Health & Productivity Revitalizer®

Published by
Healthy Ideas Press
P.O. Box 541
Greenwood, TX 76246 USA
orders@saveherlife.com
http://www.saveherlife.com

Unattributed quotations by Mellanie True Hills

ISBN 0-9766008-0-3

Library of Congress Control Number: 2005921152

First printing 2005
Second printing 2006

Printed in the United States of America

Cover design by Stephanie True Moss, True Moss Communications

The information in this book is not intended to be medical advice and is not a substitute for consulting your doctor or members of your health care team before making changes.

Dedication

This book is dedicated with love to my husband, Dave, and my son, Jason, and

In appreciation to my mother, Celesta True, and my sisters, Stephanie True Moss and Tracy True Dismukes, and

In memory of our dad, Howard Albert True, and our recently-departed cousin, Darlene Orton.

Many thanks. I love you all.

About the Author

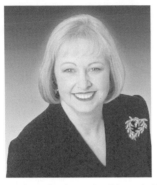

Mellanie is a heart survivor, having had a close call in emergency heart surgery. Using her second chance, she coaches individuals to create healthy lifestyles that revitalize their health, and works with organizations to create healthy workplaces that transform productivity.

As the founder and CEO of the American Foundation for Women's Health, a non-profit organization dedicated to education and awareness about women's health issues, Mellanie's mission is to spread awareness of heart disease and how to prevent it. She provides a message of hope and encouragement, sharing how to take control, decrease stress, and protect against heart disease. Audiences consistently say, "You changed my life."

Previously, Mellanie was an Internet pioneer at J.C. Penney Company, Inc., over a decade ago, where she led the creation of one of the early corporate web sites as well as an intranet and supplier extranet. At Dell Inc., she was the executive in charge of creating and executing Dell's intranet vision and strategy. At Cisco Systems, Inc., she was an eBusiness Strategy Thought Leader in Cisco's Global High-Tech Internet Business Solutions Practice where she served as a Trusted Advisor to top executives of some of Cisco's largest high tech customers.

As a renowned Internet visionary, she is the author of two intranet and groupware best-sellers, Intranet Business Strategies and Intranet as Groupware, published by John Wiley & Sons. She wrote for numerous business and technology publications, including a regular syndicated column for the Dallas Business Journal and other city business journals.

She addressed audiences of hundreds and thousands at some of the earliest Internet events, in locations as diverse as Montreal, Singapore, Rio de Janeiro, Johannesburg, and New Delhi, and has keynoted adjacent to such Internet luminaries as Tim Berners-Lee, creator of the World Wide Web. She was also a celebrity judge at the First India Internet Awards, in New Delhi, India.

In addition to being a wife and mother, Mellanie serves on the Executive Committee of the Leadership Texas Alumnae Association Board of Directors and the Executive Council of the Texas Alliance of Women's Health Networks. She is a member of Women in Technology International (WITI), the National Speakers Association (NSA), the Heart of Texas chapter of the National Speakers Association, and Mended Hearts.

She also volunteers with the American Heart Association, where she serves on the local board of directors and as a speaker and media spokesperson on their behalf.

Visit her web site at http://www.mellaniehills.com, or write her at mhills@mellaniehills.com.

Acknowledgments

I extend my grateful appreciation and thanks to the following, who have helped me in so many ways.

My family and extended family, for their patience, love, and support through my health journey and the subsequent labor of love that became this book.

Stephanie True Moss, for her beautiful cover design, her input into the book, and especially for her dedication and patience.

Clyde W. Yancy, MD, for his beautiful and articulate message in the Foreword and his graciousness in providing incredibly perceptive and valuable feedback with which to strengthen the book.

Ceil and Deborah, my friends and fellow heart disease survivors, for sharing their stories to benefit other women.

Natalie Elliott, for her guidance on my nutrition journey.

Jim Sterne, my long-time friend and mentor, who started me on the path to writing my first books and who continues to encourage me today even though my current subject matter is so far afield from our shared Web knowledge.

The many women who generously contributed to the book by sharing their experiences— Martha Alikacem, Norma Almanza, Susan Baughman, Cheri Butler, Carla Daws, Karen Hiser, Brandy Meeks, Jeanie Meyer, Jo Rake, Karlene Seime-Noble, Tammy, Vicki, Carol, and some anonymous contributors who shared even though they were unable to take credit for their contributions.

Those who took the time to review the book and provide important feedback that made this book better because of their contributions— Boyd Lyles, MD, Linda Byars Swindling, Lorri Allen, Debra Brown, Sharon Frey, Gayle Golladay, Joyce Hills, Karen Hiser, Susan Macaulay, Lisa McNew, Nina Rowan, and Claudia Snow.

Many staff and volunteers at the American Heart Association Capital Area Division and Texas Affiliate, for involving me in their mission and helping me spread the word—AHA staff, Diane McIntyre, Midge LaPorte Epstein, Mindy McReynolds, Rebecca Willms, Elizabeth Muenzler, Michelle Hutsell, Matt Danelo, Remy Morris, Stephen Brown, Brion Oaks, and many others; fellow Williamson County and Capital Area Board members, for sharing their wealth of knowledge and expertise; and fellow Heart Walk volunteers, including Stephen List and Diane Graden.

My sisters in the Leadership Texas Class of 2003, the Leadership Texas Alumnae Association, and the LTAA Board—far too many to name without risking leaving someone out—for their continuing friendship and support and for opening my eyes to new ways of thinking and new directions for my life.

Audrey Selden, for her mentoring, guidance, and example.

Many speaker friends in the National Speakers Association, especially the North Texas and Heart of Texas chapters, for supporting and propelling me forward with my mission and passion.

Media personalities who have helped get out the word about women and heart disease—Dennis and Niki McCuistion, Lori Parker, Paul Serrell, Jess Britain, Jim Cox, Bob Gourley, Jordan Rich, Cary Nosler, Raymond Francis, Liz Gunderson, Hedi Headley, Ken Johannessen, Rachel Lehcar, Dr. Nancy Loft, Paul Morgan, Tim Quinn, Wendy Wiese, and Bill Wilkerson.

Many people at corporations, agencies, and associations who have so warmly embraced my message.

Many wonderful colleagues and others from whom I've learned and grown and whose guiding hands have shaped my path.

Thank you all.

Foreword

In early 2005 [as this book went to print], it was reported that heart disease lost its place as the leading cause of death in America for persons under the age of 85 to cancer. Based on the latest reliable data [from the year 2002], there were 476,000 deaths due to cancer and 450,000 deaths due to heart disease. It is encouraging that deaths due to heart disease are falling but nearly half a million Americans are still dying from a largely preventable illness and it is apparent that more awareness of risk factors, more adaptation of prevention strategies and earlier implementation of effective treatments for heart disease are urgently needed. This need is particularly acute in the female population. The misnomer that women succumb more frequently to diseases other than heart disease must be overcome as heart disease does not respect gender and women can be tragically victimized by heart disease. This book by Mellanie True Hills chronicles a real life story of a remarkable woman struck by heart disease and the resultant rally of her human spirit that led to a restoration of her health.

As a survivor of heart disease, Mellanie True Hills has written a sensitive, personal, witty and informative account of her struggle with heart disease and the journey that she has experienced towards renewed health. Using her unique perspectives acquired in the business world along with the passion generated in the acknowledgment that women remain largely unaware and/or ill-informed about heart disease, she has researched an impressive repository of information on heart disease and has crystallized the HEART program designed especially for women. Her HEART program emphasizes a heart-healthy diet, regular exercise, stress reduction, appropriate time for rest and rejuvenation and a positive and forward thinking attitude about health. These messages are timely, accurate and are conveyed by Mellanie in a warm vernacular that brings the reader into the story as participant, perhaps even as a confidante, and not as an insulated observer. I have met Mellanie. Her message is sincere; her passion is palpable; and her energy level is enormous. When I listen to her, it is evident that "she gets it".

Part I of this book is all about Mellanie's abrupt wake-up call and her realization that as a middle-aged woman at the prime of her life, she had heart disease. Clearly, heart disease can strike anyone anywhere and at anytime. She chronicles not only the sterile methodical journey she faced but also the emotional upheaval that this unwelcome guest created. Part II may be entitled "What Every Woman Should Know About Heart Disease" but every man should read this section as well. The statistics she quotes are accurate and the picture she portrays of the enormity of heart disease is alarming and thought provoking. Appropriately, she includes much-needed information on stroke and raises the attention level for this debilitating disease. Chapter 10 is beautifully done and captures truly what all women should know about heart disease. Chapter 11 is succinct and definitely the right message at the right time. **Heart disease is preventable.**

Part III represents the distinguishing feature of this book. Many resources are available that will provide factual data regarding heart disease but few offer an easy-to-follow, logical and pragmatic "plan". Chapter 14 is a true gem and raises 5 questions that all should address—how many of us have ever given thought to "what would my ideal life look like?" and then to "how and when that ideal life can be attained?" These are soul searching thoughts that will recruit the requisite energy needed to adapt a plan towards better health. HEART is that plan and chapters 16-20 outline the steps required. Chapter 16 condenses much of the rhetoric about dieting into digestible statements that build towards a sensible strategy for a lifetime of healthy eating. Chapter 18 is a highlight. The references to e-mail as a source of stress and the contrast between morning and night people are both humorous and on target. How many of us would love to have our e-mail in-box vaporized?! The book finishes with steps to take towards taking control of one's life.

In reading this book, don't miss the personal testimonies from many woman interviewed about their own struggles with heart healthy living. The inclusion of many aphorisms, especially those authored by remarkable women, gives this book a very intimate appeal.

As a cardiologist, researcher, educator, writer and volunteer, I know firsthand what the toll of unchecked risk factors for heart disease can be. Over the last 15 years I have witnessed the personal despair, disruption of families, and loss of happiness that premature disability and death due to heart disease and stroke can cause. But I have also witnessed and participated in the explosion of information and treatments that can and do make a difference. Technology and innovation have yielded clever devices, safer surgeries and dramatically effective medications to treat heart disease. Despite our success in treating heart disease and stroke, no treatment is better than optimum health. The best treatment for heart disease is prevention. Attaining optimum health is a long and challenging journey and like any challenging journey, the hardest part is the first step. This book and the HEART Program represent a great first step. I highly recommend this to all who want to reduce their risk of heart disease and stroke.

Clyde W. Yancy, M.D.
Professor of Medicine
Director of the Cardiovascular Institute, St. Paul University Hospital
Medical Director of the Heart Failure/Heart Transplantation Program
University of Texas Southwestern Medical Center
American Heart Association National Physician of the Year 2003
Dallas, TX

Contents

Figures

Introduction

Wisdom comes from learning from others' mistakes and not repeating them. Why am I writing this book? So that you can learn from my mistakes.

Are you speed-obsessed? Do you live an overstressed life in this 24-by-7, do-it-now world? Are you constantly in multitask mode, instant messaging in meetings and conference calling while driving? Are you on a productivity treadmill? I was.

This "always-on" lifestyle put me at risk for a heart attack or stroke. It could do that to you, too. You may think that you're too young for that, or not at risk. That's what I used to think. I wish that someone had told me the things contained in this book before I almost died from heart disease. Now I have heart disease forever.

This guidebook will help you to know what to do when you encounter the blinking red warning lights of your health, and more importantly how to avoid having heart disease sneak up on you. We will explore what you can do to prevent heart disease, or at least to decrease your risk of it. We'll talk about what puts you at risk, what you can easily change, and what you can't, what to look for, and what to discuss with your health care provider.

I have made this book easy to read so that it's something you can read on a plane flight, sitting in the departure lounge, waiting in the doctor's office, or after the kids go to bed and you're exhausted from your day because I know that those are about the only places or times that you have time to read.

In this book, my purpose is not to tell you how to live, or what to think; my purpose is to provide you with facts, information, and tools to decide on the approach that is best for you. You're unique, and one size never fits all, so this guidebook is full of tools and processes to help you think about your journey and to create a plan to save your own life. I'll share with you my HEART program that may be valuable for your own plan.

I wrote this book for you, so you can avoid what I've been through. In Part I, we'll focus on my story, and the lessons learned from it, and throughout Parts II and III, we'll focus on what you can do to prevent heart disease and other serious illnesses, with a few relevant experiences of mine sprinkled in. Along the way, we'll learn from the experiences of others as well. Here's what we'll cover on our journey together.

Overview of the Book

Part I: Surviving the #1 Killer
Gives you background about the problem, shares my story, and discusses what you can learn from it.

> Chapter 1: It Kills More Women
> Chapter 2: My Story: One Millimeter to Live
> Chapter 3: My Program to Save My Life
> Chapter 4: Getting a Second Chance
> Chapter 5: Heart Disease is Forever

Overview of the Book

Part II: What Every Woman Should Know About Heart Disease
Gives you the information for figuring out how this impacts you and what you can do about it.

Chapter 6: Heart Disease is the #1 Killer of Women (and Men, Too!)
Chapter 7: Heart Disease Risks
Chapter 8: Heart Attack and Stroke Symptoms
Chapter 9: Diagnosing Heart Disease
Chapter 10: Why is Heart Disease More Difficult to Diagnose in Women?
Chapter 11: Heart Disease is Preventable

Part III: Designing Your Plan to Save Your Own Life
Gives you information to prevent heart and other diseases, and helps you implement your plan to save your own life.

Chapter 12: Why You Need a Plan
Chapter 13: The Process for Developing Your Plan
Chapter 14: Where Do You Want to Go?
Chapter 15: Creating Your HEART Program
Chapter 16: Healthy Eating: How I Lost 85 Pounds and You Can Lose, Too
Chapter 17: Exercise Daily
Chapter 18: Attitude About Stress: How You Can Learn to Love Stress
Chapter 19: Rest, Relaxation, and Rejuvenation
Chapter 20: Take Proactive Control of Your Health
Chapter 21: Putting It All Together and Making a Commitment

Appendices

Appendix A: Master Forms
Appendix B: Resources

Figure I.1: Overview of the Book

As you learn what you can do, please take the time to pass along this information to others. Please share it with the other women in your life—daughters, sisters, cousins, friends, and business colleagues. You can help save the lives of all the women you love.

When you finish this book, you'll have new ideas and a plan for taking back control of your own life and increasing your health and longevity. When you've finished the book, please e-mail me (HEART@saveherlife.com) to let me know about your plan and how it's going. I want to help you on your journey to a lifetime of good health.

Thanks for joining me on this journey. Let's get started.

Part I: Surviving the #1 Killer

Although the world is full of suffering, it is full also of the overcoming of it.
Helen Keller, 1880–1968, Educator

It Kills More Women

It's shocking! Heart disease kills more women than men in the US and has for twenty years. Why haven't we heard that? How could we possibly lose almost half a million women each year in the US to cardiovascular diseases (heart disease and stroke) and not be hearing about it? That's almost 1,400 women every day, ten times as many as we lose to breast cancer, and five times as many as to all cancers combined. Forty per cent of us—two out of every five women—will get, and die from, cardiovascular disease. If you have a family history of heart disease, your risk is very high.

Until recently, women rarely encountered heart disease before the age of 65, and it was thought that estrogen provided a protective effect before menopause. Now, heart disease has become a younger woman's disease, often happening in our 30s, 40s, or 50s, just like with men, because there are more women in the workplace now and we have the same stresses as men at work. The impact of those stresses on us may be greater because the business world is built on a masculine model, and isn't always "female-friendly".

In addition to our stress from the business world, we tend to have family stress, as well, since women have long tended to carry a disproportionate share of the family responsibility. Though that's changing in many households, we still have the long-term effects.

What's really scary is seeing heart disease now among women in their 20s, and even in their teens. It is largely attributable to diet and overweight, especially given today's high levels of soda and junk food consumption.

Another problem is our sedentary lifestyles. With increased job demands and family needs, it's often hard to find time for exercise and taking care of ourselves.

There are many other reasons that we lose more women than men, and we'll explore those in more detail in later chapters.

Let's next explore my story—what happened, why, and most importantly what it means to you.

A wise man should consider that health is the greatest of human blessings,
and learn how by his own thought to derive benefit from his illnesses.

Hippocrates, 460 BC–377 BC, Greek physician

Chapter

2

My Story: One Millimeter to Live

What Happened to Me

March 25 was my own personal September 11. Before that, I felt immortal.

At the time, I was a road-warrior, traveling as much as 95% of the time as a consultant for a high-tech firm. A typical week meant one, two, or three cities, with marathon meetings, constant conference calls, and working around the clock. The productivity meter at work ratcheted higher every month, every quarter, and every year, and my life was frenetic and stressful. Keeping up in my field was impossible due to the relentless waves of information constantly crashing over me, threatening to wash me away. I had learned to control it, but it was still stressful.

Though I loved my job, and really did enjoy the travel, the changes caused by September 11 had made the constant travel much more stressful.

One afternoon, I was headed to San Jose for customer meetings. After running the security gauntlet, I was in the departure lounge checking e-mail and logged into a virtual meeting when a customer called.

"Hey, Rick. Sure, I'll e-mail you the latest slides when I get to San Jose tonight."

Just then, the gate agent, with her nasal voice, announced the flight. "Ladies and gentlemen, flight 1733 is ready for boarding," she said. "All Advantage Gold, Platinum, and Executive Platinum passengers are welcome to board. If the other two of you will wait a moment, we'll call for you shortly." Then she cringed as she stepped over to the door to process the herd.

As regulars on that flight, everyone wanted to get on first to stash their stuff, so I wondered if there would still be space in the overhead when I got on. Fortunately, there was, so I hoisted my rollaboard into the overhead, put my computer bag under the seat in front of me, and started pulling out my PC.

This American Airlines flight between Austin and San Jose is called the "Nerd Bird" because it has more electronic gear per-capita than any other flight. We typical geek and geekette road warriors carry a cell phone or two, a pager, a PDA, noise canceling headphones, a DVD player, a laptop PC with wireless card, a power plug for the under seat outlets, and of course enough cables to wire the terminal. The flight is so quiet—all you hear is the tap, tap, tapping of keyboards.

Why do we techies carry all that gear? Well, you have to work the entire flight to keep up with your job. Before we took off, I connected my PC to the wireless in the terminal and downloaded the slides for my customer.

It was a good flight, and I got a lot of work done. I worked on several presentations and meeting agendas, and also processed many of the hundreds of e-mails that had come in while I was in meetings all day.

When we landed, I turned on my cell phone, pulled my rollaboard out of the overhead, plunked my computer bag on top, and charged up the jetway. This time something was different as it was harder to breathe. "Maybe it's molds from the recent rains here in San Jose," I thought, since I'm very sensitive to molds.

I kept on going through the terminal, past security, down the escalators, and out to the rental car shuttle, which had moved about two blocks farther down. As I slung my bags on board, I could barely breathe and my left shoulder ached. I thought back to that USA TODAY article I had just read containing new research that women have different heart attack symptoms from men—where men have crushing chest pains, which they frequently refer to as "the elephant on the chest," and buckets of sweat, women's symptoms are more subtle.

If our symptoms are so subtle, how does a woman know that she's having a heart attack? She can have any, or all, of the four main symptoms: shortness of breath, tiredness (or fatigue or sleeplessness), nausea, or pain in the left shoulder or arm (or jaw or shoulder blade). I had two of those symptoms, so I arranged to see my doctor when I arrived back in Austin, and monitored myself the rest of the trip.

I told my doctor that I had experienced shortness of breath, which I chalked up to molds, but wondered if it could be related to my heart because I also had pain in my left shoulder. She decided to do a chest X-ray and an EKG—the EKG was abnormal so she sent me straight to the emergency room.

"Can I drive myself?"

"No," she answered, "Can someone else drive you, or should I call you an ambulance?"

Fortunately, my husband was close by, and he took me to the emergency room. On the way, my blood pressure spiked. It had been low at the doctor's office, but I guess I was just scared and panicky. Wouldn't you have been, too?

At the emergency room, they took me straight to the Trauma Center and treated me for a heart attack. There were half a dozen doctors and nurses running around, asking questions, poking and prodding, and giving me nitroglycerin—it was enough to give you a heart attack!

When the cardiologist arrived, his gentle demeanor put me at ease. He ordered chest X-rays, scans, and all kinds of tests, but didn't find anything. He felt that it wasn't a heart attack, but did want to keep me all weekend for monitoring.

I was a reluctant patient. I had a lot of thoughts going on in my head. I didn't want to be in the hospital for the weekend—I needed to be home working on my taxes as it was almost April 15 and with all my traveling I hadn't had the time to do them. While I was in the emergency room waiting to get checked into a room, I returned customer calls—I had promised I would call them back after my doctor appointment. I wasn't really worried about what they would find in monitoring me—I'm too young for heart disease.

As you can tell, it hadn't sunk in. I was totally in denial. I didn't understand the significance. Do you ever feel that way? Do you ever postpone taking care of your needs because you're so busy? We women tend to do that because we're always taking care of everyone else.

"I'll go home and get your suitcase," my husband said.

"You'll need to unpack all of my business suits since I just got home, and please be sure to bring my computer."

When he got back without my computer, I was really annoyed. I had so much e-mail and work to do that I just couldn't get by without it. But he refused to bring it. What could I do? I resigned myself to spending the weekend reading. At least he brought travel books so I could focus on planning the trip to Rome and Florence. At least I could do something useful, and not totally waste my time!

Can you relate to that? Never wanting to waste a minute? While a road warrior lifestyle is stressful, being a Type A meant that some of my stress may have been self-inflicted. Where did this Type-A behavior come from? I think mine was genetic. While I grew up, my mother was a high-achiever who could never tolerate idle hands. Type-A behavior now seems to run in our family. Does it run in your family, too?

All weekend they monitored me, and on Monday we were to meet with the cardiologist to decide between a stress test and a heart catheterization. A stress test indicates heart problems, but isn't very reliable. A more reliable alternative is the heart catheterization. Doesn't that sound like fun? To do it, they cut open your leg, pump in some dye, and X-ray you to look for blockage. A catheterization is 100% reliable, but is invasive. I didn't want to do it, and I sure didn't want to be railroaded into it.

On Monday morning I couldn't have coffee or food just in case I needed the catheterization. I was groggy and walked up and down the hall to wake up. Suddenly, my cardiologist zoomed in holding up a printout.

"What were you doing?" he asked, wide-eyed.

"Just walking," I innocently answered.

"Well, you just had your stress test," he said. "We're doing that heart catheterization now."

Larry, the orderly, wheeled me down. He was a hoot! He wore teal, yellow, and lavender printed scrubs—quite a contrast to his flaming red hair. He cracked killer jokes. As he wheeled me out the door, I asked "Is this a joke? Where are we going?"

"The mobile cath lab," he said, as we bumped down the sidewalk and across the parking lot, laughing and joking. Then he strapped the gurney into a window-washer platform, and I'd swear I saw him hoist me up by pulling on ropes.

Once inside, Beth, my bartender, knocked me out and before I knew it we were done. I came to as they wheeled me back into the hospital. They had found that a major coronary artery was 95% blocked, and I was probably within hours of a heart attack. It was such a relief to have escaped that!

The next day, they would send me to their sister hospital for a balloon angioplasty to open the blockage and metal scaffolding, called a stent, to keep it open. It's just routine, so there was nothing to worry about.

I knew that I would miss some meetings, so that evening I set about making phone calls, leaving voicemails, rescheduling meetings, and asking colleagues to cover for me, all the while thinking that I would be back at work within a day or so and back to San Jose for very important customer meetings early the next week. There was so much to be done that I really couldn't afford to be gone.

The next morning, the paramedics transported me to the other hospital. I remember them asking me what I did, and when they found out that I was a road warrior with a high-tech company, they started grilling me about how to set up Internet and wireless access and all kinds of techie subjects. We laughed and joked the whole way, alleviating much of my anxiety. Since they weren't familiar with the route between the two hospitals, and I drove it frequently, I pointed out landmarks and directed them to the hospital while lying down strapped to the gurney. "You drive," one of them jokingly suggested.

At the other hospital, the cardiovascular surgeon popped in to meet me. He was tall and olive-skinned, with a strong accent and a very serious demeanor. My husband and I grilled him extensively about the procedure, his experience, and anything else that was relevant as I absolutely wasn't going under until both my husband and I were confident about this. He had lots of experience, and a great track record, so there was nothing to be concerned about.

As they wheeled me into the operating suite, I chatted and laughed with the nurses until the surgeon arrived. They gave me local anesthesia. I remember being awake through the entire procedure, and watching it on the TV monitors above me. I kept hearing seriousness in the surgeon's voice, but couldn't quite comprehend what it meant. He seemed to be having difficulty. I heard him say, several times, "It's too short. Get a longer guide wire. We need one more millimeter."

Even after removing the original guide wire, and replacing it with the longer one, he still seemed to be having difficulty, but I couldn't really tell what the problem was. When we were done, I could see that he was pale and ashen gray and was hunched over.

After he left, the surgical team seemed to be having trouble stopping the bleeding, but finally they succeeded in stopping it.

Once they got me back to my room, I noticed that the nurse kept coming in at what seemed to be unusually frequent intervals. My blood pressure was dropping to dangerously low levels, to the point where they had to call the surgeon that evening. Fortunately, my husband recognized that I was dehydrated, probably from fasting and surgeries two days in a row. Once I got some water, my blood pressure started to rise and eventually returned to normal.

My husband seemed quite worried and upset, but I didn't know why—it wasn't until the next morning that I learned of what the surgeon had told him.

The next morning, when the surgeon came in, he asked, "How are you doing this morning?" There was no hint in his voice of the challenges the day before. "Yesterday was difficult. Your blockage was at a juncture," he said, as he drew a picture of it. "It was close—putting the stent here at the blockage, in just one side of the juncture, would have cut off blood flow to the other. You almost had a massive heart attack right there on the operating table. It was close, but one millimeter made all the difference." It was then that I realized that even though he had performed over a thousand successful stent procedures, he had nearly lost me.

"If you don't do something about your weight, your stent will need to be replaced, probably within three to six months," he continued, with his tone extremely serious. "After that close call, we can't do another angioplasty, so you'll have open heart surgery." That hit me hard and just about knocked me flat.

"Let's get you out of here. You can go back to work in a few days, but don't travel for at least two weeks." With that, he reached over and pulled off one of my heart monitor leads and said with a grin, "that'll get a nurse in here quickly," as he displayed his less-serious side.

One millimeter made all the difference. One millimeter is barely visible to the eye, and yet, it saved my life.

Why It Happened

What caused my heart disease? You can't prevent it if you don't know what causes it. More importantly, how can you avoid it?

It's odd. I really wasn't a candidate for heart disease. I'm much too young—that's an older person's disease, or so I thought. The reality is that you can be vulnerable at almost any age.

There are four major risk factors: smoking, diabetes, high blood pressure, and high cholesterol, which I didn't have any of. In fact, my blood pressure and cholesterol were low as I always ate healthfully, with mostly organic foods and no fried foods. Did I have family history? At first, my doctors thought so, but have since discounted that, too.

It boiled down to my being overweight and over-stressed. Stress hijacks healthy habits, and caused me to be overweight.

However, stress and overweight weren't really the causes of my heart disease—they were just symptoms. As I probed deeper, I realized that I was so busy with the craziness of my road-warrior life that I hadn't taken care of me. I thought I had, but there was so much more I could have done. Now I have heart disease forever.

Health is worth more than learning.
Thomas Jefferson, 1743–1826, US President

Chapter

3

My Program to Save My Life

I was extremely grateful for getting a second chance, so I have made changes as a result.

As I mentioned, my cardiovascular surgeon told me that if I didn't make big changes, my stent would fail and I would be back for open-heart surgery. I had to get myself under control. To do so, I created my HEART Program, which you'll learn more about in Part III.

Here are the first three areas I focused on, based on my doctor's mandate:

1) Diet

2) Exercise

3) Stress management

Diet

Though I already ate mostly organic foods, with lots of fresh fruits and vegetables, and didn't eat fried foods, my doctor still mandated that I go on a fat-free diet. I had to lose weight immediately to reduce my risk, so I resigned myself to my fate. I simply had to get used to it, whether I liked it or not.

They started me on a fat-free diet in the hospital, and the fat-free milk there was so disgusting that the organic fat-free milk at home actually tasted good. I guess my body gave me some extra help in adjusting to it.

I've now learned that it's not such a bad thing after all, and I don't really miss the fats. Foods seem to taste fresher and healthier, though perhaps my brain just has me fooled. I have lost weight and I feel much better, so the fat-free diet has been a good thing.

Exercise

My doctor insisted that I get more exercise, at least 30 to 60 minutes every day, and strength training, when possible. The exercise would increase the good cholesterol, cause me to lose weight, and reduce my stress.

Stress Management

Stress was my demon, and that was the most difficult change to tackle. I couldn't do it overnight—it was going to take time.

When I first left the hospital, my doctor insisted that I take a few days off from work, and not travel for the first two weeks, and once I resumed traveling, I would have to be sure that there was a good hospital nearby.

My first day at home, I took it easy by working in my home office for only about 10 hours of e-mails, phone calls, and catching up on work. Does that sound familiar? It was actually quite therapeutic, though, as I spent time catching up with colleagues and customers, and didn't do anything that I didn't want to do. I was stunned, though, to receive flowers and gift baskets from customers and colleagues.

When I returned to full time work a couple of days later, the first thing I did to get my stress under control was to start taking back control of my life. No more working around the clock. I pushed back on demands, and started saying "no" more often.

I started researching heart disease in women, and what to do to avoid it happening again. It was then that I created the basis of my own plan for recovery and how to take control of my life and health, which I call my HEART Program. That plan is detailed in Part III.

When I started back to traveling two weeks later, I went to the airport early to walk for an hour instead of working. On the plane, I wasn't as fanatical about work and e-mail, stopping often to enjoy things that I didn't pay attention to before. For example, one evening, I raised the window shade of the plane just in time to watch the most glorious sunset over the Grand Canyon—a priceless view that I'll never forget. In fact, I set a goal then to go see the Grand Canyon up close, which we just did.

One challenge I faced in traveling, and in daily life as well, was a residual issue from the hospitalization. After being tethered to the IV for 5 days, I ended up with a frozen shoulder, and also experienced some nerve damage to my hand during the hospitalization, so I underwent many months of physical therapy to return my arm and hand to normal use. Can you imagine the challenge of hoisting a rollaboard and computer bag on and off of the rental car shuttle with just one working arm? I learned a lot through this temporary disability. I managed, with pain, and with occasional help from kind souls. I had always been very independent, but I learned that you don't have to be independent and self-sufficient to travel.

Another part of taking control of my stress was to ensure that we took frequent vacations, starting immediately. We hit the open road as a family in our motorhome, getting away from it all, with no e-mail or cell phones. When possible, the whole family went on my business trips. It's much more relaxing to take the motorhome on the open road rather than flying. It takes longer, but I use the time to write and reflect. It's the best think time.

Finally, when exercising, instead of multitasking by listening to tapes, I let my mind wander to de-stress.

Chapter

4

Getting a Second Chance

As I got myself under control with diet, exercise, and stress management, I started learning more by researching the problem and finding potential solutions.

Just three weeks after leaving the hospital, I attended my second session of Leadership Texas, a program for Texas women. As I shared my experience, and talked about how women have different heart attack symptoms from men, some of my classmates were motivated to do something about their own health. At subsequent sessions, many told me about being checked out, and even having catheterizations that found blockages. From that, I realized that I was given a second chance so I could spread the word and help other women avoid heart disease.

Many women don't know that heart disease is the number one killer of women, and believe that breast cancer is our number one risk. Only recently has the medical field even come to recognize that women are just as vulnerable to heart disease as men. With our subtle symptoms, by the time we recognize them, it may be too late. That is why we lose more women than men.

I realized that women's symptoms are easy to dismiss, both by women and by their doctors, and that without raising awareness, we will continue to lose many more women. We're frequently tired, which can mean that we're not getting enough exercise, but it can also be a symptom of heart disease. Sleeplessness can be related to menopause or hot flashes, but can also be a symptom of heart disease.

As I got myself under control, I volunteered to speak for the American Heart Association and became truly passionate about helping others prevent heart disease. But I knew that there was something more that I needed to do.

For years, I had thought that when our son was grown, I would spread the word among parents about dealing with major allergies in kids. It's about that time, but I wasn't sure how to transition from Internet and e-business consulting to health. But as I reflected following my own health issues, it was as though God was saying, "Did I get your attention finally?" Yes, I'm paying attention now.

But how could just one person make a difference against such a huge killer, one that takes a million people each year in the US alone? If I could make a difference for just a few people, it would be worth doing. But how?

As I was soul searching, I thought back to a few years earlier when I was a consultant and decided that I wanted to write a column for the Dallas Business Journal. I wrote that down on a yellow sticky note and stuck it on my computer monitor, where every day I would focus on it. Within that same week, at a meeting of the National Speakers Association, I introduced myself to the woman seated behind me who happened to be the publisher of the Dallas Business Journal. When she heard that I had just written two Internet-related books, she asked "Would you be willing to write a CyberSense column for us?" That's how I came to have a Dallas Business Journal column.

I decided to make the leap, having faith that, as before, the answers would appear when I needed them. I hoped that by sharing my story I could save you, and many other women, from heart disease and other serious illnesses. I created a plan, and made the leap from my road warrior job. Even though I loved the job, this was so important.

I'm especially focused on women because we have so much stress in our lives, putting us at risk. Are you under stress? What woman isn't? We have lots of stress in our lives because of all the different hats we wear.

Stress-related illnesses, especially heart disease and stroke, are costly in human terms, health care costs, and lost productivity. Since cardiovascular diseases account for the lion's share of company and individual health care costs, the return on investment from making these changes is huge. I now write articles and books, coach individuals in creating healthy lifestyles and managing stress, and work with organizations to create healthy, productive workplaces. Together we can stop this insidious killer.

Chapter

5

Heart Disease is Forever

Once you have heart disease, you have it forever and are more at risk for related issues. You also can't get individual medical coverage; I know, because I've experienced it.

About six months after my original heart problems, I experienced another heart issue. I had just returned from our girls' getaway to Italy, involving 24 hours of travel to get home. Just a few days later, I flew to San Jose on business—out one evening, and back the next. Twelve hours later, I was sitting at my desk doing e-mail.

"It felt like my heart stopped," I told my husband. "I'm dizzy, so I'm going to lie down on the couch."

I was wearing shorts, and he noticed that one leg looked different from the other. "Your right leg is pale, and it feels cold below your knee," he told me.

"It feels numb, and my foot feels like pins and needles. My right eye seems fuzzy, too," I told him.

The doctor told us to rush to the emergency room, where they would be waiting for us.

I had multiple blood clots, or perhaps a single clot that broke apart and went to my right leg and to my right eye. My cardiologist said that I was very lucky as most clots go to the brain as a stroke.

This was caused by atrial fibrillation—a quivering of the upper chambers of the heart. I'm now on a beta-blocker for the atrial fibrillation and on a somewhat challenging blood thinner, Coumadin®, to prevent further clots. But, overall, I got off easy. I've since had other atrial fibrillation incidents, but for now, it appears to be under control.

I've since learned that if you're susceptible to heart problems, your risk of blood clots increases sixteen-fold on plane flights of 6 hours or more. You've probably read about "economy class syndrome", or deep-vein thrombosis (DVT). My clots were different— arterial, not vein clots, but if you're susceptible, it really doesn't matter. A blood clot can kill you, or give you a stroke.

I'm obviously susceptible as both incidents happened just after a flight. For now, I'm grounded, and haven't flown in months. I even got a call from the executive offices at American Airlines saying, "We just wanted to find out why you're not flying with us any more since you used to fly about 100,000 miles per year with us. Are you mad at us?" No, but flying could have killed me.

Unfortunately, I haven't seen anything to indicate how you might know that you're at risk from flying. However, some clues may be found in research done by the University of Dresden Medical School in Germany. They found that passengers on flights of eight hours or longer were twice as likely to develop blood clots. Of 964 passengers studied, 27 (3%) developed blood clots. One third of those had deep-vein thrombosis (DVT), and the rest had smaller clots that dissolved on their own. All who developed clots had risk factors—overweight, age 45 or over, family history of blood clots, cancer, recent surgery, or were on the pill or hormone replacement therapy.

I flew for years, even lots of long international flights, with no troubles. However, at the time, I wasn't overweight (a recent occurrence), wasn't on hormone replacement therapy, and wasn't over 45. Those are risk factors to keep in mind if you fly long flights.

As we end Part I, let's explore some of the lessons about women and heart disease that were my motivators for telling you my story. If this could happen to me, when I didn't really have the risk factors, other than being a Type A, it can happen to anyone, especially if you're a Type-A woman.

1) **Women's symptoms are subtle**, and are different from men's symptoms. Pay attention to your body—what you don't know, or don't act upon, can hurt you, or even kill you. Take proactive control of your health now.

2) **Life changes may be necessary** to save your life. It's better to change now, as you may not get that second chance.

3) **Heart disease is forever**. Once you have it, it's too late, and puts you at risk for more problems.

As we move into Part II, we'll look at what every woman should know about heart disease, and some facts about other related issues as well.

Part II: What Every Woman Should Know About Heart Disease

Many persons have a wrong idea of what constitutes true happiness.
It is not attained through self-gratification but through fidelity to a worthy purpose.
Helen Keller, 1880–1968, Educator

Chapter

6

Heart Disease Is the #1 Killer of Women (and Men, Too!)

Let's explore some facts about the impact of heart disease.

In the US, heart disease and stroke are the #1 and #3 killers, each year taking nearly one million people, and accounting for almost 40% of all deaths.

In Figure 6.1, you can see that heart disease and stroke, the cardiovascular diseases (CVD), take nearly twice as many lives as all cancers combined. These numbers are for both men and women in the US, and are similar throughout the world today.

Deaths by Cause (000s)

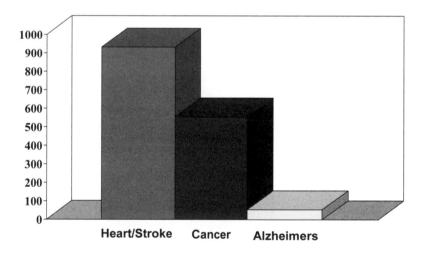

Figure 6.1: Deaths by Cause in 2001, Source: National Heart, Lung, and Blood Institute

The numbers for women for heart disease and stroke in the US are particularly startling. Most of us don't know that two out of every five women—forty per cent of us—will have cardiovascular disease, and die from it. In just the US we lose 1,400 women every day to it—wives, mothers, sisters, daughters, co-workers, and friends. Many never had any symptoms.

Here are some significant heart disease and stroke facts for the US, though the numbers for the rest of the world are similarly shocking. These numbers come from the American Heart Association (AHA) and the National Heart, Lung, and Blood Institute (NHLBI) of the US government's National Institutes of Health (NIH).

1) Contrary to widespread belief, heart disease is the #1 killer of women, and stroke is #3, together taking nearly 1,400 women per day. That's over half a million women every year.

2) Each year, 1.2 million Americans have a heart attack.

3) One out of every two women can expect to have heart disease and to die from it.

4) Forty per cent of all women's deaths today are attributed to heart disease and stroke.

5) Women account for more than sixty per cent of stroke deaths.

6) Heart disease kills more women than men, and has each year for the past 20 years.

7) Heart disease and stroke kill ten times as many women as breast cancer, and more than all cancers combined. Cancer survival rates are increasing, but many of those cancer survivors will die from heart disease.

8) Women have different heart attack symptoms from men, and they're more subtle. Many women, and their doctors, don't know this.

9) Many women don't know that they have a heart problem until AFTER they have had a heart attack, making death the first symptom for many women.

10) Men are much more likely than women to survive heart attacks, and to get more aggressive treatment for their heart disease. As a result, 38% of women who have heart attacks die within one year.

11) In addition to being the number three killer, stroke is the number one cause of long-term disability, with survivors experiencing memory loss, vision problems, and paralysis. Almost five million Americans are stroke survivors, with almost thirty per cent of them permanently disabled.

One of the most shocking global statistics comes from a Columbia University estimate that by 2030, 41 per cent of deaths among those ages 35–64 in the developing world will be due to heart attacks, strokes, and diabetes compared to only 12 per cent for the same age group in the US.

This is all so frightening, and is why I'm so motivated to find ways to change this.

Let's end this chapter by recapping some important facts about heart disease and stroke. In Figure 6.2, I've recapped facts for the general population of women.

Heart Disease and Stroke Facts for Women

- ❑ Heart disease and stroke are the #1 and #3 killers of women in the US
- ❑ For the past 20 years, they have killed more women than men
- ❑ Account for 40% of women's deaths, more than the next five causes combined
- ❑ Responsible for ten times as many women's deaths as breast cancer, and twice all cancers combined
- ❑ Currently 20% of US women have cardiovascular disease, and the numbers are growing
- ❑ After menopause, risk of heart disease increases 2–3 times
- ❑ Of women who died suddenly, 63% had no prior symptoms
- ❑ Heart disease risk increases with physical inactivity, which is more prevalent among women

Figure 6.2: Heart Disease and Stroke Facts for Women, Source: American Heart Association—2003 Update

African American and Hispanic women are at even greater risk. Here's a recap of the statistics for African Americans in Figures 6.3, and for Hispanics in Figure 6.4.

Heart Disease and Stroke Facts For African Americans

- ❑ African American women are at greater risk–39.6% vs. 23.8% for Caucasian women
- ❑ African American males and females are at greater risk for heart disease and stroke, and have higher death rates.
- ❑ At higher risk because
  - o 55% are physically inactive
  - o 77% are overweight
  - o 21% smoke
- ❑ High blood pressure is a leading cause of stroke
- ❑ Heart disease risk increases with physical inactivity, which is prevalent in the African American population

Figure 6.3: Heart Disease and Stroke Facts for African Americans, Source: American Heart Association—2003 Update

Heart Disease and Stroke Facts for Hispanics

- ❑ Leading cause of death for Hispanics
- ❑ Responsible for 33% of deaths in Hispanic women
- ❑ Cardiovascular disease rate is 27%
- ❑ High blood pressure is a leading cause of heart disease and stroke
- ❑ At higher risk because
  - o 57% are physically inactive
  - o 72% are overweight
  - o 12% smoke
- ❑ Heart disease risk increases with physical inactivity, which is prevalent in the Hispanic population

Figure 6.4: Heart Disease and Stroke Facts for Hispanics, Source: American Heart Association—2003 Update

*In the business world, the rearview mirror
is always clearer than the windshield.*
Warren Buffet, 1930– , Financial Executive

This rearview mirror philosophy applies to us, too.
Mellanie True Hills

Chapter

7

Heart Disease Risks

Risk Factors

We have explored the statistics surrounding heart disease and stroke, and you're probably wondering what causes them. Therefore, let's explore the factors that put you at risk.

Recent research has confirmed that the majority of heart attacks are due to the Big Four risk factors:

1) Smoking

2) Diabetes

3) High blood pressure

4) High cholesterol

There are, however, four other important risk factors:

5) Family history

6) Overweight

7) Inactivity

8) Stress

We'll discuss these eight risk factors in detail below.

For many years, age and gender were considered to be risk factors as well—men were considered more at risk, especially after age 45; women weren't considered at risk, at least not until after age 55.

The thinking is changing—heart disease and stroke are now equal opportunity diseases. Women today are more at risk of dying than men, but not specifically because of our gender. It is because our symptoms are different, and doctors are relearning what they thought they knew about heart disease and gender.

We're also seeing shifts in age, with younger and younger people having heart attacks and strokes, largely due to the eight risk factors. As we age, our risk does increase, but it is more a factor of our other risk factors than of our age.

Let's dive in and look at the eight important risk factors, and in Chapter 11, we'll explore what you can do about these risk factors.

Smoking

Smoking is the number one risk factor. If you smoke, STOP NOW!

My friend, Deborah, recently had open-heart surgery related to smoking, with high cholesterol and stress as other risk factors. She was only 42 years old. She was kind enough to share her story with us, in Figure 7.1 below.

Deborah's Story

Deborah is in marketing, and was under a lot of stress. Back in the fall of 2002, she first experienced some symptoms that she now attributes to her heart. She felt tightness in her chest when she was walking. Her doctor diagnosed her with allergy related asthma—not considering the possibility of heart problems in a young woman with no family history.

The following spring, as her symptoms worsened, Deborah began thinking it was heartburn because taking an antacid made the symptoms go away. It wasn't until 2003 that her symptoms could no longer be dismissed. Driving on the freeway on her way to a business meeting, she began experiencing chest pains. Thinking it was indigestion, she reached for an antacid, but was unable to find them. The pain continued to worsen and didn't dissipate as usual. Almost panicked, and without a cell phone handy, Deborah looked for public areas to pull over and ask someone to call 911.

Then, as quickly as the pain had started, it finally stopped. Deborah proceeded to her meeting and conducted business as usual. When her immediate tasks were complete though, Deborah realized just how shaken up the experience had left her. She called a co-worker that was a former nurse, and who advised her to go to the ER. There, the doctors determined that she had not had a heart attack, but they wanted to keep her overnight to run some tests. She was on a deadline at work, and wanted to go home to get her laptop, but the doctors wouldn't even consider it.

The next day, her nuclear stress test indicated a problem. They needed to do a heart catheterization the next morning. In it, they found a 95% blockage in her left main artery, and took her straight from the catheterization to emergency bypass surgery. Here she was, just 42 years old, having had open heart surgery.

Deborah's risk factors were smoking, high cholesterol, and stress at work due to a relatively new job for which she had relocated to a new city. While she knew that smoking could cause lung cancer, she didn't know of the strong correlation between smoking and heart disease. In looking back, she feels that if she had known about the connection between heart disease and smoking, she probably would have quit smoking much sooner. And, if she had it to do over again, she would have started on cholesterol medication sooner.

She has quit smoking, and does cardiovascular workouts and watches her diet, but recovery from heart bypass is a long, long journey.

Deborah's Story

And she, too, has learned that heart disease is forever, as a few months after her bypass surgery, she had to go back in for a stent to open up another 95% blockage in her right main artery.

Deborah shared with me her thoughts and recommendations for you and other women. Women need to pay close attention to managing their stress, using techniques such as guided imagery, sound therapy, and alternative medicine. She suggests making self-care the number one priority, and cautions us to always listen to our bodies. Most importantly, don't let your doctor dismiss your symptoms. If necessary, find a new doctor. And, if you're in a bad situation—get out, because it's not worth your life or your health. These are important suggestions from someone who has been there.

Figure 7.1: Deborah's Story

A recent study, done at New York's Presbyterian Hospital, found that women who smoked were more likely than men to develop lung cancer, even though they both smoked the same amounts. Does this hold true for heart disease? We don't know, but why risk it?

Smoking doesn't just cause heart disease and lung cancer. In announcing a recent Centers for Disease Control report, the US Surgeon General announced that this new report "documents that smoking causes disease in nearly every organ in the body at every stage of life." In addition, he mentioned that smokers typically die 13 to 14 years earlier than nonsmokers.

Even if you don't smoke, you may still be at risk from second-hand smoke from cigarettes, cigars, or pipes. Did you know that second-hand smoke is the third leading cause of preventable death in the US, and that passive smoke can have just as devastating an effect on you as actually smoking? Just two hours of exposure to smoke, such as in a smoke-filled club or at work, can increase your heart rate and lead to a heart attack. Secondhand smoke doubles your risk of heart disease. Of the 440,000 Americans who die each year from smoking-related illnesses, approximately 35,000 are nonsmokers who die from heart disease caused by secondhand smoke. Shockingly, secondhand smoke leads to ten times more heart disease deaths than cancer deaths.

Diabetes

Diabetes is a disease where the body is unable to use its most important fuel source, glucose from foods, because of a problem with insulin, the hormone in the body that utilizes glucose. Diabetes happens when either the body doesn't make enough insulin or when it can't properly utilize the insulin it makes.

Diabetes is also a very important risk factor for heart disease as high levels of blood sugar and insulin can damage the heart and the blood vessels. Diabetics are from two- to four-times more likely to develop heart disease than others, and are more likely to die from a heart attack. In fact, two out of every three diabetics will typically die from cardiovascular disease, but fortunately new medical interventions are changing that, as mentioned below.

The number of diabetics is rising rapidly, having increased by forty per cent over the 1990s, and is thought to be due to the rapid increase in overweight and obesity, as defined later in this chapter. A recent study by doctors from Harvard found that increased consumption of corn syrup, coupled with decreased consumption of fiber, parallels the increase in Type 2 diabetes, a form of diabetes that typically occurs in adults.

About 18 million Americans now have diabetes, which can also lead to adult blindness or kidney failure. Many Americans with diabetes are currently undiagnosed. The US Department of Health and Human Services estimates that about 41 million American adults between the ages of 40 and 74, about 40% of the US adult population, have pre-diabetes. They also estimate that one in three children will develop diabetes. African Americans and Hispanics have the highest rates of diabetes. Studies have also indicated that diabetes is a much more serious risk factor for heart disease in women than it is for men.

Another scary statistic related to diabetes is the recent finding correlating Alzheimer's and diabetes. Diabetics are 65 per cent more likely to develop Alzheimer's, and many who don't develop Alzheimer's do develop dementia.

There is great news for diabetics, however, from a new study that found that cholesterol-lowering statin drugs can significantly reduce the risk of heart disease in diabetics. The American Diabetes Association's newest Clinical Practice Guidelines for doctors (http://www.diabetes.org) recommend that about 99% of diabetics over age 40, those with total cholesterol of 135 or more, should be on statins. These same guidelines also recommend that diabetics keep blood pressure under 130/80, get cholesterol under 200, maintain blood glucose levels (A1C test) at 7% or less, and take aspirin.

High Blood Pressure

Do you know your blood pressure? Is it normal? I recently read that about one-third of US women have blood pressure readings that are too high. Could that be related to the stress in our lives?

Until recently, we were told to keep our blood pressure below 140/90, but that has changed, with the current guidelines recommending 120/80, or below. Blood pressures between 120/80 and 140/90 are now considered *prehypertensive*, meaning that hypertension (high blood pressure) is a strong future possibility. For those over age 50, the top number (systolic pressure) is more important as a risk factor than the bottom number (diastolic pressure).

About fifty million Americans, and one billion people worldwide, have high blood pressure. Why is blood pressure such an issue? Primarily because high blood pressure can indicate possible plaque buildup in the arteries. Plaque consists of soft fats or hard calcium that gets deposited in the arteries and builds up, much like rusty pipes, narrowing the arteries and diminishing blood flow. The narrowing of those arteries causes the heart to work harder to pump blood through the smaller vessels, producing higher pressure.

Therefore, having high blood pressure puts you at increased risk for a heart attack, heart failure, stroke, or even kidney failure. The American Heart Association reports that if you have *uncontrolled* high blood pressure, you are three times more likely to get heart disease, and seven times more likely to have a stroke.

Even scarier is that for those with high blood pressure, cold weather further increases the risk. A new study that was reported on at the 2004 European Society of Cardiology meetings in Munich (http://www.escardio.org/) indicated that those with hypertension are at increased risk of a heart attack due to changes in weather. For example, when temperatures drop below 39.2 degrees, the number of heart attacks doubles for those with hypertension. In addition, any day that the temperature dropped nine degrees or more, regardless of how cold it was, heart attacks among hypertensives also increased. Why? Because cold weather constricts the blood vessels.

African Americans and Hispanics have increased propensity toward hypertension, as do kids. Incredibly, up to two million kids in the US have hypertension, especially in the most vulnerable groups. For example, the Medical College of Georgia studied high caffeine consumption in teens and found that African American teens experienced a fourteen point increase in their blood pressure from drinking three or more soft drinks per day over just a three day period. Wow! That's why programs such as the one put in place by the Texas Department of Agriculture, which mandates removal of soft drinks and other nutritionless foods from schools, are so important for kids' health.

If you have high blood pressure, be aware that doctors at the Mayo Clinic recently found that high blood pressure often indicates high cholesterol as well.

High Cholesterol

Cholesterol is a waxy substance found in the bloodstream and cells. It is necessary for the body to function properly, such as making cell membranes. You can have too much of a good thing, though, and that's where the problems come in. Cholesterol comes from two sources–what you eat, and what your body makes naturally in your liver. Your body makes enough, so you don't need to supplement it with diet.

Dietary cholesterol is what your body gets from the foods that you eat. It comes from animal-based foods, such as meat, dairy products, poultry, and seafood. Egg yolks are especially high in cholesterol, with one egg being almost an entire day's maximum recommended cholesterol intake of 300 milligrams. Dietary cholesterol can also raise your blood cholesterol level. Plant-based foods, such as grains, nuts, and vegetable oils, don't contain cholesterol.

Do you know your cholesterol numbers? Most people don't, so don't feel badly if you don't know them. Has your doctor suggested checking your cholesterol? Knowing your cholesterol numbers is as important as knowing your blood pressure. You should know not only your total cholesterol, but also its three components. Let's explore all of those.

Total Cholesterol

Your total cholesterol should be under 200. If it's over, your doctor will certainly want to measure the individual components. That's not a bad idea, even if your total cholesterol is below 200. The three cholesterol components are:

- Bad cholesterol (LDL, which stands for low-density lipoprotein)

- Good cholesterol (HDL, which stands for high-density lipoprotein), and

- Triglycerides

These detailed numbers provide a better indicator than your total cholesterol.

I've seen recommendations that knowing your total cholesterol number is sufficient until about age 40, and that you should then have a blood screening that tells you your HDL, LDL, and triglyceride levels. With heart disease affecting younger and younger women, I'd think that if you have any of the other risk factors, or have any concerns about it, you should discuss this with your doctor to determine whether it is advisable to go ahead and check all of these cholesterol components. It's just a simple blood test. It requires fasting, usually after midnight the night before, but that's such a small price to pay for having this very important information.

As you can see in Figure 7.2, the optimal cholesterol readings are total cholesterol of less than 200, triglycerides of less than 150, LDL (bad) cholesterol of less than 130, and 70 for heart patients, and HDL (good) cholesterol of greater than 50 for women and 40 for men.

Optimal Cholesterol Readings	
Measure	Optimum Reading
Total Cholesterol	Less than 200
Triglycerides	Less than 150
LDL (Bad) Cholesterol	Less than 130, and 70 for heart patients
HDL (Good) Cholesterol	More than 50 for women (40 for men)

Figure 7.2: Optimal Cholesterol Readings

LDL (Bad) Cholesterol

Too much LDL cholesterol in your blood leads to a build-up in the artery walls, forming plaque, a thick, hard substance that causes atherosclerosis, more commonly known as "clogged arteries." Clots forming nearby can then block blood flow to the heart, causing a heart attack, or block blood flow to the brain, causing a stroke. That's why LDL is so bad.

The AHA recommends keeping your LDL cholesterol below 130, with 100 being optimal. If you already have heart disease, you need to be below 70.

Can you get your LDL cholesterol too low? Apparently not, as the current recommendation is to go as low as you can. A recent study reported that patients on a particular statin had median LDL levels of 62, compared to 95 for those on a different statin. The lower LDLs correlated with a 16 per cent lower rate of heart disease and stroke, and a 28 per cent lower death rate. The lower the LDL cholesterol, the better. Recent research has pointed to statins lowering our risk of many cancers as well.

While some cardiologists have joked that we should put statins in the water, apparently that's not so far-fetched as Britain allows statins to be sold over the counter, with no prescription required.

In some cases, your doctor may order a special screening to break LDL into its components. Before my surgery, my cholesterol numbers were fine, but we wondered if one of the LDL components was out of line but was being masked by the other LDL components. My cardiologist subsequently ordered a "Berkeley Panel" to separate out the various LDL components, but those numbers, too, were fine.

Even if your numbers are fine, don't go around eating fats with reckless abandon. Even with great cholesterol numbers, you still should be cognizant of any other risks that you may have.

HDL (Good) Cholesterol

Where LDL cholesterol is bad, HDL cholesterol is good. A normal HDL reading for women is 45–60, and for men, 35–50.

HDL's role is presumed to be to move cholesterol from the arteries to the liver so that it can be removed from the body. There's even a belief that HDL may remove cholesterol from plaques already built up in the arteries, helping protect against heart attack. When you don't have enough HDL, the body keeps building plaque in the arteries.

Smoking, being overweight, and lack of exercise, will keep your HDL levels depressed, putting you at more risk. My doctor said that exercise is the best way to increase my HDL level, and that I should be walking briskly 30–60 minutes every day. Some studies have also indicated that you can increase your HDL cholesterol through moderate use of alcohol. Moderate is the operative word here.

Triglycerides

Triglycerides are a form of fat that comes from food. Though high triglyceride levels are often correlated with heart disease, having high triglycerides doesn't automatically mean that you will have heart disease. High triglycerides are often found along with high total cholesterol, high LDL, and low HDL, the combination of which does put you at risk.

Some recent news on the exercise front indicated that ten-minute workouts are more effective in lowering triglyceride levels. Researchers at the University of Missouri–Columbia found that three ten-minute workouts were more effective in lowering triglyceride levels than one thirty-minute workout. However, they only tested for triglyceride levels, so this may not apply to the other cholesterol components. One physician commented recently that anything less than 30 minutes at a stretch doesn't improve the HDL cholesterol, so longer stints of exercise still appear to be necessary.

Other Problems Related to Cholesterol Levels

As if this isn't already enough to make us pay attention to our cholesterol levels, one new related data point is that women with higher bad LDL cholesterol levels tend to have lower bone densities. A woman with an LDL of 160 or higher has twice the risk of osteopenia, a precursor to osteoporosis, than a woman with a normal LDL of 129 or less.

Finally, as if we needed any more reasons to control our blood pressure and cholesterol, a study done at the University of California at San Francisco found that middle-aged participants who had multiple heart disease risk factors among the Big Four (smoking, diabetes, cholesterol, and hypertension) were twice as likely to develop dementia in old age as those with only a single risk factor. Having all four risk factors tripled the risk over study participants without any risk factors.

Family History

Do you have a family history of heart disease? Has anyone in your family had a heart attack? Have several family members died from heart disease, or did anyone die at a young age from it? Did you have a close male family member (grandfather, father, or brother) who had heart disease before age 55, or a close female family member (grandmother, mother, or sister) who developed heart disease before age 65?

This is a risk factor that you can't control, and is therefore important and valuable information for helping your doctor to decide what health screenings to order and when to start doing them. This doesn't just apply to heart disease; your doctor should know about family members with cancer, diabetes, osteoporosis, and a host of other possible illnesses. One of my doctors said that this is the most important information that a patient can provide her.

Over the past year or so, there have been studies that have isolated specific mutations of genes that definitely cause heart attacks, and discoveries of others that seem to confer a protective effect, even in those with high blood pressure, high cholesterol, or other heart risks. Another new study has found that African Americans are more likely than European Americans to have gene variations linked to heart attacks, which could help explain the fact that African Americans appear to be more vulnerable to heart disease.

These research findings open up the possibility that one day we could have genetic testing that would tell us more about our level of risk. From that, we could take the necessary steps to deal with the findings. But until then, it's best to presume that we need to do whatever we can to minimize our risk.

Overweight

The facts continue to roll in about the effect that being overweight has on your health. Carrying around extra weight is a tremendous strain on your heart. This hits very close to home for me as it was one of my two risk factors.

If you're overweight, you're at increased risk for heart disease and stroke because being overweight stresses your heart and can cause high blood pressure. You're also more at risk for diabetes, a major risk factor for heart disease.

The statistics shown in Figure 7.3, about the percentages of the US population that are overweight, are pretty shocking.

Overweight and Obesity (see Figure 7.5) Among Americans Age 20 and Older	Women	Men
Non-Hispanic White	57%	67%
Non-Hispanic Black	77%	61%
Mexican	72%	75%

Figure 7.3: Overweight and Obesity Among Americans Age 20 and Older, Source: American Heart Association

Please keep in mind that when I use the terms *overweight* and *obese* in this book, I'm talking about the official clinical classifications from the National Heart, Lung, and Blood Institute, which we'll explore over the next few tables. It doesn't mean that if you weigh a few pounds more than what you would like to weigh that you're automatically at risk.

How can you know if you are overweight? Let's explore this question using the guidelines from the National Heart, Lung, and Blood Institute (NHLBI), which are reproduced in Figure 7.6. The guidelines classify overweight based on Body Mass Index (BMI) and Waist Circumference. Let's first define BMI, and then we'll put it all together.

Body Mass Index

Body Mass Index (BMI) is an estimate of body fat. The easy way to find out your BMI is to go to the BMI Calculator at the web site of the National Heart, Lung, and Blood Institute (http://nhlbisupport.com/bmi/) and enter your height and weight (select the American or metric measurements tab.)

Alternatively, you can select the "Go to BMI Tables" link on that page. To use the table, look up your height in inches by moving down the left column, then go across that row to your approximate weight, and then look up the column to the heading, which tells you your BMI.

In Figure 7.4 are the official categories for various BMIs, which you'll see again in Figure 7.6.

Weight Description Using BMI	
Weight Description	BMI
Underweight	Less than 18.5
Normal Weight	18.5–24.9
Overweight	25–29.9
Obesity	30 or more

Figure 7.4: Weight Description Based on BMI, Source: National Heart, Lung, and Blood Institute

To give you a sense of what these numbers really mean, I've provided, in Figure 7.5, the height and weight combinations at which a woman has a BMI of 25, classified as **Overweight**, a BMI of 30, **Obesity**, and a BMI of 40, **Extreme Obesity**. For example, if a woman is 4' 10" tall and has a weight of 118 pounds or less, her classification is normal; if 119–142 pounds, overweight; if 143–190 pounds, obesity; and if 191 pounds or more, extreme obesity.

Women's Weight Classifications			
Height	Weight (pounds)		
	BMI=25 Overweight	BMI=30 Obesity	BMI=40 Extreme Obesity
4'10" (58)	119	143	191
4'11" (59)	124	148	198
5' 0" (60")	128	153	204
5' 1" (61")	132	158	211
5' 2" (62")	136	164	218
5' 3" (63")	141	169	225
5' 4" (64")	145	174	232
5' 5" (65")	150	180	240
5' 6" (66")	155	186	247
5' 7" (67")	159	191	255
5' 8" (68")	164	197	262
5' 9" (69")	169	203	270
5' 10" (70")	174	209	278
5' 11" (71")	179	215	286
6' 0" (72")	184	221	294
6' 1" (73")	189	227	302
6' 2" (74")	194	233	311

Figure 7.5: Women's Weight Classifications, From National Heart, Lung, and Blood Institute's Body Mass Index Table (http://www.nhlbi.nih.gov/guidelines/obesity/bmi_tbl.pdf)

Waist Circumference

Waist circumference, which measures abdominal fat, is the other important factor in determining the overweight classifications. Simply measure your waist with a tape measure.

Figure 7.6 shows the National Heart, Lung, and Blood Institute's table for classifying overweight and obesity by BMI and Waist Circumference, and also indicates the level of risk for cardiovascular disease, hypertension, and Type 2 diabetes that is associated with each category.

Classification of Overweight and Obesity by BMI, Waist Circumference, and Associated Disease Risks

Weight Description	BMI (kg/m²)	Obesity Class	Risk of Type 2 Diabetes, Hypertension, and Cardiovascular Disease	
			Women 35 in (88 cm) or less	Women >35 in (88 cm)
Underweight	< 18.5		–	–
Normal	18.5–24.9		–	–
Overweight	25.0–29.9		Increased	High
Obesity	30.0–34.9	I	High	Very High
	35.0–39.9	II	Very High	Very High
Extreme Obesity	40.0+	III	Extremely High	Extremely High

Figure 7.6: Classification of Overweight and Obesity by BMI, Waist Circumference, and Associated Disease Risks, Source: National Heart, Lung, and Blood Institute (http://www.nhlbi.nih.gov/health/public/heart/obesity/lose_wt/bmi_dis.htm)

In Figure 7.6, a woman with a waist measurement of 35 inches or more (the far right–hand column), combined with a BMI of 25–29.9 (in the second column from the left), is listed as being *overweight* (first column), and therefore is at high risk (far right-hand column) of diabetes, hypertension, heart disease, and stroke. A BMI of 30–34.9 is categorized as *obesity*, and has a very high risk if the waist circumference is 35 inches or more. As you see, the higher the BMI, the higher the risk.

Being overweight or obese may be one of the most important risk factors for women as the Harvard Nurses Health Study found that about 30 percent of women's heart attacks were correlated with being overweight or obese.

Of course, adding in any of the other risk factors discussed in this chapter increases the risk even more.

Even if a woman has a waist measurement of less than 35 inches, she is still at increased risk if her BMI exceeds 25. Even with a normal weight, having a waist circumference of 35 inches or more puts a woman at higher risk due to having an apple shape.

You've probably heard that you're more at risk if you're apple-shaped, meaning that you carry your excess weight around your waist, rather than if you're pear-shaped, where you carry excess weight in your hips or thighs. That is true—being apple-shaped indicates that you are more at risk. The reason is that fat on the hips is stored just under the skin, whereas fat at the waist is stored deeper, frequently surrounding the internal organs, which is much more dangerous.

We women tend to be more pear-shaped until after menopause, and then we start to store our excess fat around our waists. That's when our risk increases. If you have an apple-shape, you may have what's called "metabolic syndrome"

Metabolic syndrome is defined as having three, or more, of the following five conditions: obesity (typically abdominal fat), high blood sugar, high blood pressure, high triglycerides, and low HDL (good) cholesterol. About one-fourth of adults have metabolic syndrome, which puts them more at risk for heart disease, stroke, diabetes, and cancer. In fact, a study of metabolic syndrome found that those with it were from three to four times as likely to die of a heart attack.

In addition, eating lots of fats, especially saturated fats and trans fats (discussed in detail in Chapter 16), further increases fat accumulation in the waist area, and increases the risk.

While apple vs. pear is an important heart-health distinction, be aware that many nutrition authorities say that body shape has nothing to do with your nutritional needs, contrary to what you might read in some diet books.

Weight is becoming a huge health problem in the US and around the world. Where in 1986 only one in every 200 Americans was extremely obese, by 2000 that had more than tripled to one in every 50. Obesity-related deaths are expected to overtake tobacco-related deaths in the near future.

The Centers for Disease Control classifies deaths in the US based on the original source of the problem, as shown in Figure 7.7. Death from heart disease can be due to tobacco, obesity, or a number of other causes. While tobacco was the top cause, obesity was a very close second, and was up more than 100,000 from the prior decade. Obviously, by 2010, it will have well overtaken tobacco.

Cause Of Death in the US in 2000	
Cause	Number Of Deaths (Per Cent Of Total)
Tobacco	435,000 (18%)
Obesity	400,000 (17%)
Infectious disease (pneumonia and flu)	75,000 (3%)
Car crashes	43,000 (2%)

Figure 7.7: Cause of Death in the US in 2000, Source: Centers for Disease Control, US Department of Health and Human Services

Correlation of Overweight with Other Diseases

Overweight and obesity have been correlated with other diseases and health issues as well.

- American Cancer Society research has shown that postmenopausal women who had gained 21–30 pounds over their weight at age 18 were at a 40% greater risk of getting breast cancer than those who had only gained 5 pounds or less. It's thought that breast cancer risk increases due to the excess fat tissue increasing the body's estrogen levels.

- That same 20 pounds or more of weight gain also increases your risk for Alzheimer's. Women in their 70s who were overweight by at least 20 pounds had an increased risk of having Alzheimer's in their 80s. For each increment that their BMI went up, their risk of dementia increased by 36%. Researchers theorize that this is due to decreased blood flow to the brain and heart.

- Women with a waist circumference of 35 inches or more were two and a half times as likely to get cataracts, a leading cause of adult loss of vision, as those with a waist circumference of 31.5 inches or less.

- Obese men have twice the risk of colon cancer, and obese women (BMI=30 or more) face two-to-four times the risk of breast cancer and endometrial cancer. Fat around the abdomen seems to be more reactive, leading to faster cell growth, including growth of cancerous cells.

Inactivity

A sedentary lifestyle probably goes hand-in-hand with being overweight, so you can eliminate two risk factors by just getting up and moving. Just like any other muscle, if you don't exercise it, your heart will atrophy. You've got to get your heart pumping at least 5 times a week. Cardio workouts, such as a brisk walk, are important for overcoming this risk factor.

High Stress

Whether or not stress actually causes heart disease has been very controversial, but I believe that it does due to two data points.

1. Many of the heart attack survivors that I have interviewed for another book didn't have the classic risks factors, but many did have high stress.

2. A study of 43,000 Japanese women done by the University of Tsukuba found that those who were very stressed were one and a half to two times as likely to die of stroke or heart disease, even though they tended to be five years younger. We don't know whether this study translates to other races and nationalities, but we do know that African American women have the highest death rate from heart disease, and it is theorized to be due to their bodies producing less nitric acid, which the body uses to handle stress by opening up the blood vessels to maintain blood flow.

As I was finishing the editing of this book, Canadian researchers at McMaster University reported their findings at the 2004 European Society of Cardiology conference in Munich. Those findings should quell any disbelievers.

In the study, the factors accounting for almost 90 per cent of all heart attacks were isolated. Number one was abnormal cholesterol, as measured by a new test, ApoB, which you will learn about in Chapter 9. That accounted for almost half of the heart attack risk. Smoking was next, at thirty-six per cent, followed by diabetes, high blood pressure, and abdominal obesity.

One of the biggest surprises for the researchers was that stress and depression came in sixth, followed by insufficient fruits and vegetables and inadequate exercise. Thus, we're finally getting research confirmation that stress really is a factor in heart attacks.

In other studies presented at the European Society of Cardiology, two studies found that exposure to air and noise pollution significantly increased heart attack risk, largely due to the increase in stress hormones released by the body. Another study, which I mentioned earlier, found that the risk of heart attacks doubles during cold weather for those with high blood pressure, and again, stress appeared to have been a contributor.

Of course, stress is now being implicated in many other diseases as well. We will explore stress in much more detail in Chapter 18.

My friend, Ceil, is a heart survivor, and stress was a factor with her heart. She was kind enough to let me share her story with you, in Figure 7.8 below.

Ceil's Story

Ceil is in law enforcement, a very stressful field. Back in 1995, she was in New Orleans, with her husband while he attended a convention. She decided to do touristy things. As she took a plantation tour one day, she felt tired, a little bit sweaty, and out of breath. She came back exhausted, and went to sleep.

The next day, she felt achy, with chest congestion, almost like she had the flu. She could barely pack to go home, and needed to sit down to catch her breath.

While flying home, she felt severe chest discomfort, but it was NOTHING like the classic pressure or tightness or the proverbial 'elephant on the chest.' That evening, when she got home, her husband rushed her to the hospital emergency room. Blood tests there revealed that she probably had a heart attack while they were changing planes in Houston. The doctors did an angiogram (catheterization), and found that a small artery had closed off. They inserted a balloon, though the artery was too small for a stent.

Ceil really had no early warning of problems, other than an unusual EKG the previous year, but the cardiologist didn't find a thing.

A month after her surgery, she had some stomach and chest pains, which were said to be reflux. She also developed asthma, and would wake occasionally gasping for air.

Then, in 2000, during her regular cardiologist visit, she commented that it felt like she had butterflies fluttering in her chest. They did a stress test, which was abnormal, and decided to do another angiogram. The situation was so serious that they had to do a triple bypass. This time, she never actually had chest pains, or any other symptoms, besides the butterflies.

Like most bypass survivors, Ceil's worst pain was in the breastbone where they had to crack it open to reach the heart. The entire first year she was in constant pain, and finds the area occasionally still painful four years later. Recovering from bypass is a long journey.

Ceil's Story

She now pays lots of attention to the things that were the causes, with stress and being a Type A among the main ones. She also feels that she could have done some minor diet adjustments—she knew she needed to for general health, but ignored it. Like most heart survivors, she now notes every unusual ache or pain, just in case.

When I asked Ceil what she would recommend for other women, she suggested that we all need to do our homework, reading up and becoming knowledgeable about our health. But don't believe everything you read on the Web—consider the source and their motives. Also learn to listen to your own body telling you things, even if you don't understand them. It's generally trying to get your attention before it's too late!

Figure 7.8: Ceil's Story

Other Risks

There are other risks to consider in special cases.

For example, women who have been through menopause tend to be more at risk, particularly if the menopause resulted from a hysterectomy that removed the uterus and/or ovaries. Until recently it was thought that hormone replacement therapy had a protective effect on our hearts, but two recent US government-funded studies have refuted that theory.

You're also more at risk if you have had a chronic disease, such as heart disease, stroke, cancer, or other.

- If you have had a heart attack or stroke, you're more at risk for a second one.

- If you have atrial fibrillation, a quivering of the upper chambers of the heart, you're more at risk for blood clots that can cause a stroke.

- Some cancer drugs have been correlated with increased risk of heart attacks. Though we don't exactly know why, the statistics are starting to point out this relationship.

- Sickle cell anemia, a genetic disorder among African Americans, causes clots that can cause a stroke.

If you have any of these, which are risks you can't avoid, you should be scrupulous about avoiding the risks that you can.

Risk Assessment

Now that we know about risk factors, let's assess your current health and potential risks. Consider your own personal level of risk for each of the following, in the table in Figure 7.9, below.

1)   Smoking

2)   Diabetes

3)   Blood pressure

4)   Cholesterol

5)   Family history

6)   Overweight

7)   Activity level

8)   Stress

9)   Other risks/measures

You can find a copy of Figure 7.9 in the master forms section, Appendix A, which allows you to keep all of your exercises together in one place. As you fill out this exercise and others, feel free to do them in the master forms.

First, enter your age and gender.

Then, under the column labeled Current, just fill in your current state for each risk (i.e., smoking, yes or no) or the appropriate measure(s) of health, such as blood glucose (if you're diabetic), blood pressure, cholesterol, height, weight, BMI, and waist circumference, if you know them. If you're reluctant to write down any of these numbers (such as weight), that's OK—just think about them in your head without writing them down.

If you don't know all the answers, just fill in what you do know, but don't stop just because you don't have all the answers. For any categories in which you don't know your numbers, such as blood pressure or cholesterol, just treat them as potential risks for now and revise them later when you get your actual numbers. By taking your plan with you for your next doctor visit, having them listed as potential risks will jog your memory to discuss them with your doctor.

In section 9, Other, list any chronic conditions or measures that you track that are important to your health, and fill in the current or recent numbers. For some people, some of the other blood tests we'll discuss in Chapter 9 may be important. For me, since I'm currently on Coumadin®, a blood thinner, my International Normalized Ratio (INR), a measure of my blood's clotting ability, is one of the most critical numbers for me. I would list my latest INR readings under Other.

In the column marked Normal/Ideal is the currently-regarded normal level for each measure, at least in the US, as recommended by various guiding organizations. These include the American Heart Association, American Diabetes Association, and the National Institutes of Health's National Heart, Lung, and Blood Institute.

In the column labeled Risk Y/N, indicate No if your measure is within the acceptable range, or Yes if your measure puts you at risk.

Finally, in the column labeled Risk Count, put a check mark or an X for those categories that you marked with a Yes, and count the total number of risk factors that you have. We'll use this information in Chapter 15 to figure out how to deal with these risks.

Risk Assessment				
Risk Factor/Measures	Current	Normal / Ideal	Risk Y/N	Risk Count
Age _____				
Gender _____				
1. Smoking	_____	No_____	___	___
2. Diabetes	_____		___	___
Blood glucose	_____	7%, or less_____		
3. Blood pressure	_____	120/80, or less____	___	___
4. Cholesterol			___	___
Total	_____	Under 200_____		
Triglycerides	_____	Under 150_____		
LDL (Bad)	_____	Under 130, or under 70 in heart patients		
HDL (Good)	_____	Over 50_____		
5. Family history	_____	No_____	___	___
6. Overweight	_____		___	___
Height	_____			
Weight	_____	See Figure 7.5_____		
BMI	_____	Less than 25_____		
Waist circumference	_____	Less than 35 inches_		
Weight classification	_____	Normal_____		
Risk (BMI & waist)	_____	See Figure 7.6_____		
7. Activity level	_____	Moderate to active__	___	___
8. Stress	_____	Controlled/managed_	___	___
9. Other risks/measures			___	___
_____	_____	_____		
_____	_____	_____		
_____	_____	_____		
Total Risks				___

Figure 7.9: Your Risk Assessment

In the next chapter, we will explore heart attack and stroke symptoms.

A clever person solves a problem. A wise person avoids it.
Albert Einstein, 1879–1955, Physicist

Chapter

8

Heart Attack and Stroke Symptoms

What is a Heart Attack?

There are two kinds of events that most people think of as heart attacks. One, the myocardial infarction (MI), is a true heart attack, whereas, the other, Sudden Cardiac Arrest, is often caused by a heart attack.

1) Myocardial infarction (MI) occurs when fatty plaque builds up in an artery and then eventually ruptures or bursts, spawning a blood clot that blocks the artery and starves the heart muscle of oxygen.

2) Sudden Cardiac Arrest happens when the heartbeat effectively stops, which is generally caused by a myocardial infarction. When death results, it is called Sudden Cardiac Death (SCD). Sudden Cardiac Arrest used to be fatal. Now, if an Automated External Defibrillator (AED) is used within four-to-six minutes, there is a 50–75% chance of survival. Many lives have been saved by AEDs, including several middle school students in the Pflugerville school district here in Austin because AEDs are available in all district schools. As a member of the local board of directors of the American Heart Association, I endorse AHA's programs that are driving placement of life-saving AEDs in all public places.

Women's Heart Attack Symptoms Are Different

How do you, as a woman, know if you are having a heart attack?

While men typically have crushing chest pain—the elephant on the chest—most women don't experience this. Where men often generate buckets of sweat, described as having warm Gatorade poured over them, women don't typically have this symptom either.

Women, in contrast, often have subtle, silent symptoms. Figure 8.1 shows the heart attack symptoms most frequently mentioned by women—shortness of breath, tiredness or fatigue, nausea or mild heartburn, or pain in the left shoulder, arm, jaw, or shoulder blade. While I experienced shortness of breath and pain in the left shoulder and arm, several of the women heart attack survivors I've interviewed mentioned that nausea or mild heartburn were their only symptoms. While men typically have very similar sets of symptoms, it's obvious to me from my interviews that each woman has her own unique set of symptoms, or in some cases, just one symptom.

Most Common Heart Attack Symptoms Mentioned by Women
1. Shortness of breath
2. Tiredness or fatigue
3. Nausea or mild heartburn
4. Pain in the left shoulder, arm, jaw, or shoulder blade

Figure 8.1: Most Common Heart Attack Symptoms Mentioned by Women

A ground-breaking study of women's heart attack symptoms was published in November, 2003, in Circulation, the Journal of the American Heart Association. The study was led by Jean C. McSweeney, a professor of nursing at the University of Arkansas. She and her study colleagues interviewed over 500 women heart attack survivors, who ranged in age from 29 to 95. The results are shown in Figure 8.2.

Top Twelve Symptoms Women Reported in the Month Before and During Heart Attacks	
Before Heart Attack	**During Heart Attack**
1. Unusual fatigue (71%)	1. Shortness of breath (58%)
2. Sleep disturbance (48%)	2. Weakness (55%)
3. Shortness of breath (42%)	3. Unusual fatigue (43%)
4. Indigestion (39%)	4. Cold sweat (39%)
5. Anxiety (36%)	5. Dizziness (39%)
6. Heart racing (27%)	6. Nausea (36%)
7. Arms weak/heavy (25%)	7. Arm heaviness or weakness (35%)
8. Changes in thinking/memory (24%)	8. Ache in arms (32%)
9. Vision change (23%)	9. Heat/flushing (32%)
10. Loss of appetite (22%)	10. Indigestion (31%)
11. Hands/arms tingling (22%)	11. Pain centered high in chest (31%)
12. Difficulty breathing at night (19%)	12. Heart racing (23%)

Figure 8.2: Top Twelve Symptoms Women Reported in the Month Before and During Heart Attacks, Source: Circulation, 2003, Vol. 108, p. 2621 (November 25, 2003)

Ninety-five per cent of the women interviewed for the study remembered noticing that something didn't seem quite right within the month before their heart attacks. Typically, it was fatigue or sleep disturbance. Rarely was chest pain even mentioned, and when it was, it was usually explained as being pressure or tightness in the chest instead of pain.

Once they were having a heart attack, most women described such symptoms as shortness of breath, fatigue, weakness, dizziness, cold sweat, or nausea. Again, far fewer described chest pain as a symptom. It's obvious from the list below that if you are having unusual fatigue, sleep disturbance, or shortness of breath, you should consult your doctor right away, before it's too late.

If you are having any of the other symptoms, please take them seriously and discuss them with your doctor. While they may turn out not to be indicators of heart problems, it's better not to take that risk.

This study was done at hospitals in Arkansas, North Carolina, and Ohio, and among mostly white patients, so the results could be different for other groups of patients.

What About Stroke?

A stroke is like a heart attack, except that it happens in the brain. There are two kinds of stroke. When fatty plaques rupture and send blood clots to the brain, that's an ischemic stroke, which is the most common kind of stroke. If a blood vessel feeding the brain ruptures, that's a hemorrhagic stroke.

Just so that you're aware, Figure 8.3 lists some common stroke symptoms for women. These include sudden numbness of the face, arm, or leg on one or both sides of the body, confusion, severe headache, or trouble speaking, seeing, or walking.

Common Stroke Symptoms Experienced by Women

Sudden onset of any of the following:
  1. Numbness of the face, arm, or leg on one or both sides of the body
  2. Confusion
  3. Severe headache
  4. Trouble speaking, seeing, or walking

Figure 8.3: Common Stroke Symptoms Experienced by Women

While the risk factors associated with heart attacks also apply for strokes, realize that if you have heart disease, you're at increased risk for a stroke. I shared my blood clot story with you in Chapter 5—heart disease made me more vulnerable for stroke.

Heart disease and stroke are both extremely serious. One of the reasons we lose so many women is that we frequently wait too long before calling 911. If you think it could be a heart attack or stroke, don't wait—call for help immediately.

If I can stop one heart from breaking, I shall not live in vain.
Emily Dickinson, 1830–1886, American Poet

Chapter

9

Diagnosing Heart Disease

You now know the risk factors and the symptoms—what can you do if you have some of them? What tests can your doctor order to find out if you have heart disease or are at risk for a heart attack or stroke?

Screening Blood Tests

In Chapter 7, we talked about the importance of knowing your blood pressure and cholesterol readings. Both are important in screening for heart risk; however, about one-third of heart patients have normal cholesterol levels so something else must be going on. Fortunately, newer tests hold great promise for diagnosing the risk of heart disease.

Some of these newer tests are starting to be used and recommended by the medical community, but some are still experimental and thus are not widely available or approved. For those, even if your doctor could order them, your insurance company might not pay for them. That could change any day so we'll discuss them with the presumption that in the near future they may be valuable tools in your doctor's diagnostic toolkit.

- **C-reactive protein (CRP)** is not specific just to heart disease and stroke. High CRP levels indicate inflammation or infection that can be from heart disease, stroke, colon cancer, or many other diseases. Experts from the Centers for Disease Control and the American Heart Association recommend some limited use of CRP for testing patients who are at risk, but do not recommend it for routine screening. If you have risk factors, discuss this test with your doctor. A CRP level below *one* is low risk, between *one* and *three* is intermediate risk, and above *three* is high risk. For women, a high CRP is highly significant, especially when combined with bad LDL and HDL readings. Interestingly, nutrition plays a role—a Cooper Institute study found that taking a daily multivitamin could lower CRP levels by as much as 14% over just 6 months.

- **Homocysteine** is a chemical in the blood that occurs when the body metabolizes proteins, and which can also occur naturally. High homocysteine levels in the blood indicate a higher risk of heart attack and stroke. Homocysteine testing is done routinely.

■ **Apolipoprotein B (ApoB)** is a cholesterol component, and may be a better predictor than LDL cholesterol according to a study by the University of Texas Health Science Center at San Antonio. LDL particles range in size from large to small, with the number of small ones being a better indicator. LDL tests measure all LDL particles, whereas ApoB, as a component of the protein in LDL, measures the smaller particles. In the study, ApoB levels were more accurate predictors of risk than LDL levels, but measuring LDL is still important. While the US has not adopted ApoB, Canada's national guidelines currently do recommend it.

■ **Lipoprotein phospholipase A2 (Lp-PLA2)** is called the PLAQ Test. It measures the propensity for developing plaques in the blood vessels and for their potential to rupture. Elevated levels indicate increased risk of heart attack or stroke.

■ **Placental Growth Factor (PIGF)** looks promising, and some researchers consider it better than CRP because it is specific just to heart disease risk. It tests for the presence of placental growth factor protein, which is related to inflammation of the arteries. We don't know if this applies equally to women as we only have study results for men.

Diagnostic Tests

The blood tests above can give you a good heads up, but if you are experiencing actual symptoms, your doctor will probably rely on the following diagnostic tests.

■ **Electrocardiogram (EKG)** involves hooking you up to a machine that will monitor your heart rhythm. If the EKG picks up a problem, you'll likely be sent for a stress test.

■ **Stress test** involves getting on a treadmill and walking. You may also be hooked up to ultrasound to watch the response of your heart to stress. As the treadmill speeds up, the doctor watches how your heart responds, and will also watch what happens as your heart returns to resting. A stress test isn't invasive, but it also isn't 100% accurate in showing the condition of your heart and blood vessels. There are also nuclear stress tests, done with the injection of nuclear isotopes. If the stress test indicates a problem, your next step may be a heart catheterization. If your stress test is good, that doesn't mean that you're out of the woods since stress tests may miss more than half of those at risk. One recent study found that fifty-six per cent of those who passed their stress tests actually had significant plaque buildup, as measured by electron beam computed tomography (EBCT).

■ **Heart catheterization (angiogram)** is considered the "gold standard" for identifying blockage—it's 100% accurate, but is invasive. It involves an incision in your leg, with dye pumped in to circulate through your blood vessels. The doctor watches the circulation on a scope, and records a video of it, looking for blockages as the dye moves through your system. If there is significant blockage, a balloon angioplasty and/or stent is the usual next step, though with major or widespread blockage, coronary artery bypass surgery (CABG, also called open-heart surgery) may be better.

- **Electron beam computed tomography (EBCT)**, known as calcium scan or heart scan, takes cross-sectional pictures of the body (currently 40-slices) and detects the presence of calcium deposits in the arteries, often called "hard plaque." EBCTs are controversial for three main reasons: because insurance companies don't always pay for them ($300–$600), because calcium may actually predict plaque stability (in contrast to fat-based "soft plaque"), and because recent research raised the specter of cancer risk from repeated radiation exposure. The EBCT is considered safe for diagnostic use on selected areas of the body, but over a lifetime of elective whole-body scans the radiation exposure equals that experienced by survivors of Hiroshima and Nagasaki. If you decide to do one, please do it in conjunction with your doctor. A brand new 64-slice CT, with the first one just installed at the Mayo Clinic, has cardiologists excited about the potential to totally eliminate diagnostic catheterizations.

While there are other cardiovascular diagnostic tests, and this area changes rapidly, this gives you an overview of what you might expect and what to discuss with your doctor if you are at risk.

If You Are At Risk

If you're having the symptoms discussed in the previous chapter, please discuss them with your doctor so he or she can arrange for the right tests for you. I can't emphasize this enough—discuss this with your doctor. Please don't take matters into your own hands.

I become really concerned when I hear folks talking about going to get a scan without the involvement of their doctor. Some figure that they will just go to their doctor if something is found, or they believe they can get a less expensive scan than what their doctor would order. Some want to see the results themselves, but isn't it better to have a doctor who knows your medical history to interpret the results for you? If the scan finds a problem, how will you know the urgency of it? Some folks have actually said that they don't trust their doctors to order the right tests, or to share the results with them. I personally haven't had a doctor refuse to share my results. Your health is a partnership between you and your doctor. Maybe it's time to find a new doctor if you can't trust yours. OK, end of rant.

*Science may have found a cure for most evils but it has found no remedy
for the worst of them all—the apathy of human beings.*
Helen Keller, 1880–1968, Educator

Chapter
10

Why Is Heart Disease More Difficult to Diagnose in Women?

More women than men die of heart disease every year, primarily because it's simply more difficult to recognize and diagnose heart disease in women. Some of that relates to our subtle symptoms, the ones we discussed in Chapter 8, which makes it more difficult for women and their doctors to recognize the symptoms of heart disease.

Often, however, doctors don't even think about heart disease in women, or even expect women to be heart patients. That relates to the way many doctors were trained in medical school. As recently as 1995, one-third of primary care physicians didn't know that women were more vulnerable to death from heart disease than men according to a survey by the American Medical Women's Association. Most were taught in medical school that heart disease was a man's disease.

Early studies of heart disease labeled it as a man's disease, and stated that women rarely got it until very late in life because of the protective effect of estrogen. Heart disease was rarely seen in women prior to menopause, and after that it took many years for the damage to occur that would cause the heart disease symptoms. Therefore, most doctors didn't even think about heart disease when women discussed their symptoms.

Because we women have come late to the heart disease party, many of us don't get the kind of aggressive diagnosis and treatment for heart disease that men do. When women go to their doctors or to the emergency room, often their symptoms are dismissed and they're sent home without answers. We get far fewer diagnostic tests than men, such as EKGs and stress tests, and are less often given drugs that could save our lives. Women who experience heart attacks are less likely to receive aggressive treatment, and are less likely to be sent to the Cardiac Care Unit or Intensive Care Unit.

Women also tend to be operated on less frequently because our smaller coronary arteries make it harder for surgeons to operate on us, and when we do get an angioplasty or bypass surgery we are often older and sicker. We are also more likely to die after surgery. Once we leave the hospital after a heart attack or surgery, we are less likely to be referred to cardiac rehab programs or counseling, and less likely to participate.

But it's not just doctors that don't treat women's heart disease as aggressively. We do that to ourselves as well. Often we take longer to get to the emergency room, and can lose crucial life-saving minutes, causing women to be more likely than men to die from heart attacks. On average, most victims wait three hours before seeking help, and women typically wait longer than men. We could save thousands of women's lives if we just acted at the first signs of heart attack or stroke.

On the positive side, though, we're more likely than men to seek help and to ask questions. Our strong relationships and support systems may help protect us against heart disease. But that cuts both ways—we may also be so busy as caregivers that we don't find the time and energy to care for ourselves, and thus, the stress in our lives may affect us more significantly than it does men.

Be proactive about your health. If needed, fight for answers. What you don't know absolutely can kill you. Being knowledgeable and persistent can save your life.

If you're tired or fatigued, you could just be overdoing it or not getting enough exercise, but it could be something more serious. If you frequently experience any of the symptoms discussed in Chapter 8, please take them seriously and see your doctor. It's worth repeating—for many women, the first symptom is either a heart attack or death. That's so sad because it is preventable.

If you have any of the risk factors discussed in Chapter 7, be especially cognizant of the amount of fat in your diet, especially saturated and trans fat. We'll talk in much more detail about the subject of healthy eating in Chapter 16.

Though doctors and their women patients are becoming more aware of heart disease in women, this awareness isn't translating into fewer women's deaths. If anything, the situation is getting worse as we continue to live lifestyles that put us more and more at risk. Such lifestyle risks as increased smoking, obesity, and stress are making heart disease more and more of a younger woman's disease, so we could see more deaths instead of fewer.

Chapter

11

Heart Disease is Preventable

When we explored the heart risk factors in Chapter 7, you may have noticed that many of the risk factors are things about which you can do something. This section gives you an overview of how you can prevent heart disease through controlling each of the specific risk factors.

Several risk factors may be controlled using the same solution. For example, healthy eating is the answer to a number of these risk factors, so we will explore healthy eating in much more detail in Part III.

Smoking

It's pretty simple—if you smoke, STOP NOW! Avoid being around smoke, or in smoke-filled places. If not for you, at least do it for your family.

Surprisingly, a recent European study reported that half of smokers who had a serious heart problem or heart surgery were still smoking a year later. The American Heart Association says that it's not much different in the US. That's really hard to imagine.

While you're quitting smoking, consider whether you could benefit from taking a vitamin C supplement. The University of California at Berkeley studied smokers and people exposed to second-hand smoke and found that those who took 500 milligrams per day of Vitamin C had lower levels of C-reactive protein, indicating a decrease of up to 24% in the risk of heart disease and other diseases. This study is in the April 2004 issue of the Journal of the American College of Nutrition (http://www.jacn.org/).

Diabetes

Since the incidence of diabetes is increasing rapidly due to rising obesity, getting and keeping your weight under control with diet and exercise can go a long way toward prevention. Avoiding high consumption of corn syrup, increasing your consumption of fiber, and increasing your exercise and activity levels can help as well.

Researchers at the University of Pittsburgh found that among those who were more than 100 pounds overweight and underwent gastric-bypass surgery, the average weight loss was 97 pounds and diabetes was cured in almost three-quarters of them.

If you have diabetes and are over age 40 and have a blood pressure reading of 120/80 or more, the American Diabetes Association (http://www.diabetes.org) recommends that you decrease your risk of heart disease by taking statin drugs and maintaining blood glucose levels at 7% or less.

High Blood Pressure

If your blood pressure has been creeping up slowly, it may be related to your weight, so losing weight may bring your blood pressure back under control. Try to manage your stress, too. In the interim, your doctor may prescribe a hypertension medication to help bring your blood pressure rapidly under control.

Blood pressure cuffs for home use are quite inexpensive. By monitoring your blood pressure at home, you'll know if the reading at your doctor's office is accurate. Sometimes the stress of going to the doctor may cause it to rise. Consider keeping track of your blood pressure measurements to share with your doctor, so if you're borderline, you don't end up on unneeded medication.

The US government recommends screening kids for high blood pressure, too, starting at age three, especially since the symptoms in kids are silent.

High Cholesterol

Have your cholesterol checked on a regular basis, working with your doctor to determine the best intervals. If your numbers are too high (or your HDL is too low), you may need to get more exercise, to lose weight, or to change your die by removing certain fats and cholesterol, increasing grains, increasing fruits and vegetables, and getting healthy Omega-3 fatty acids.

I'm not pushing medications, but you may want to discuss with your physician whether taking a cholesterol-lowering statin drug makes sense for you. In addition to controlling cholesterol, statins ease inflammation (as measured by CRP) and appear to reduce the risk of colon, breast, and prostate cancers.

Here are some dietary factors that can impact your cholesterol levels:

- Saturated fats from animal products, such as meat, poultry, egg yolks, and other dairy products, are the main reason for most high cholesterol readings

- Polyunsaturated fats and monounsaturated fats reduce blood cholesterol levels

- Omega-3 fatty acids, found in fatty fish, flaxseed, olives, olive oil, and walnuts, raise your good HDL cholesterol level

- Replacing saturated fats and trans fats in your diet with healthy carbs (fruits, vegetables, and whole grains) lowers your blood cholesterol level

- Smoking lowers your good HDL cholesterol – that's a bad thing, so stop smoking

- Alcohol, in moderation, appears to increase the good HDL cholesterol, but only slightly, so this isn't an excuse to start drinking. If you drink, do so in moderation (1 drink/day for women, 1–2 drinks/day for men), and be aware that there are other risks associated with drinking. AHA doesn't recommend this as a strategy for controlling your risk, nor do I, so it's best to discuss this with your physician. My cardiologist suggested a glass of wine per day to help my heart and to lower my stress.

While diet is important for managing overall cholesterol, exercise may be the best way to raise your good cholesterol. Consider walking 30–60 minutes per day to raise your HDL levels. Keep in mind that low HDL levels may have an intensified negative effect in women.

Family History

While you can't change your family history, you can be more proactive about it. Let your doctor know so that you get the appropriate tests and are monitored at the right intervals. And most of all, if you have family history, be diligent about controlling your other risk factors. The more risk factors you have, the more likely you are to get heart disease.

Overweight

I hope by now it's obvious that being overweight is a major factor in heart disease, especially for women. It contributes to three of the top four risk factors, namely diabetes, high blood pressure, and cholesterol.

Does your doctor talk with you about weight, BMI, waist measurement, and cholesterol? Does your doctor order cholesterol tests for you and discuss implications of the findings? Has your doctor discussed your diet with you? Doctors are very busy, and often you're there for a specific problem, but consider asking for a regular physical to identify anything you need to work on to improve your health.

If the chart in Figure 7.5 indicated that you are overweight, please consider finding a way to address that. This is doubly important if you are apple-shaped and carry your weight around your waist. In Chapter 16, we'll talk extensively about diet and healthy eating, and look at various ways to avoid being overweight.

As an aside, if you're pregnant, or soon may be, recent studies have found that breast-feeding helps you reduce your child's risk of being overweight or obese.

Inactivity

Going hand in hand with weight is the necessity to get up and move. Get your heart pumping at least five times a week to take care of that heart muscle and prevent heart disease. The McMaster University study mentioned earlier found that regular exercise lowered heart disease risk by fourteen per cent. A recent study found that the heart stiffens with age, leading to heart failure, and those who were sedentary had hearts that were 50% stiffer than those who were athletic.

We'll talk much more about exercise in Chapter 17.

High Stress

Finally, since stress hijacks healthy habits, if you lead a stressful life, you need to find a way to manage that stress so that you can maintain your healthy habits. We'll discuss this much more in Chapter 18.

In spite of the statistics and information in Part II, there is no reason to live in fear of heart disease or other chronic diseases. In Part III, we'll explore together what you can do to prevent heart disease and other chronic diseases and we'll create your plan to save your own life.

Part III: Designing Your Plan to Save Your Own Life

Never eat more than you can lift.
Miss Piggy, Muppet

Chapter

12

Why You Need a Plan

You may be thinking that if she knows how to do this, how come she didn't do it for herself? Should I really listen to her? Fair enough, but you can learn from my mistakes and gather wisdom without having to experience this yourself. That's certainly the easiest way.

Looking back, what almost killed me was taking my eye off the ball. I realize now that during my past five years in high tech my job was so all-consuming that I didn't take enough care of myself. I was so busy with the job, including writing down plans and carrying them out, that I didn't take the time to create and carry out a plan for my own health. Don't be so busy working that you don't take the time to take care of yourself. Please learn from my mistakes.

One of the things that made me lose focus was the cell phone. There were constant conference calls—you had to call in from the car, the airport, walking between meetings, or wherever you were. The only time available for checking voicemail and returning calls was while driving. Where I had previously listened to tapes in the car—tapes that had kept me focused on what was most important in my life—or had taken time to contemplate, with a cell phone, work took over almost every moment, including that precious drive time. With my work squeezing out my time for me, I lost touch with what I wanted for my health and outside forces intervened.

As women, we often sacrifice our own health for the health and well-being of our families. Being caregivers means that we put others first. That's the way most of us were raised. Do you remember what they tell you when you get on an airplane? Put on your own oxygen mask first, and then help others. That's good advice for every aspect of our lives.

Based on my before and after experience, let me be your poster child for what not to do, and your pathfinder in finding the way to your own healthy life.

Many of us develop plans for most aspects of our lives. Do you have a personal financial plan? If you're an entrepreneur, do you have a business plan? If you're an employee, do you have MBOs at work? What about a health plan to save your own life? Do you have one of those? Most women don't, primarily because we don't realize that we're at risk and that we need one.

You need a plan. It's not hard to do. I'll show you how. We'll work through the process together over the next few chapters.

As they say, if you don't know where you're going, any road will take you there. But if you know where you're going, you can take the most direct route. That's what we'll work on here.

I frequently coach women who want to be healthier. We start with a plan. The good news is that once the plan is done, everything just seems to fall into place and the issues drop out of the way.

Here in Part III, we'll explore what your plan should include, and how to create one. We'll go step-by-step through the process and explore each dimension. We'll spend the lion's share of Part III focused on creating your own HEART Program for the health portion of your plan. First, let's talk about some of the things involved in creating your plan.

Chapter
13

The Process for Developing Your Plan

The process for starting your plan involves just three simple rules.

1)   Start with a blank slate—a blank sheet of paper and a blank mind

2)   Brainstorm

3)   Write down whatever comes to mind

Pretty easy? It's meant to be.

Blank Slate

Starting with a blank slate lets you begin with no preconceptions. It lets you reach down into your very core to figure out what is most important to you and to use your intuition to envision your ideal life. I recommend doing this by "going into the silence", a method I learned from one of my audiotape mentors, Brian Tracy, and which I find to be incredibly powerful. (See link to Brian Tracy resources in Appendix B.)

Going into the silence is the mind's equivalent of a blank sheet of paper. Start by turning off all of life's extraneous noises and distraction (TVs, radios, cell phones, etc.), or going someplace extremely quiet. It helps to be by yourself in a place where there are no stimuli, and no people or vehicles passing by. I usually go into the bedroom and close the door, or go out to the motorhome, where I can be totally undistracted. I tell those around me to please not disturb me unless it's urgent.

To go into the silence, get comfortably into a sitting position. Sit very, very still, shut your eyes, and turn off all of your thoughts. I do that by mentally visualizing my shutting the doorways to my mind—I visualize closing off my ears and my eyes. I sit so still that all I can hear is my breathing and my heartbeat. By clearing away the extraneous thoughts, my brain is freed up to work on the specific issue at hand.

The purpose for going into the silence is to clear your brain so that your subconscious can provide you with answers. After 60 minutes, you will come out of the silence. Write down immediately any ideas that pop into your brain. The purpose was to clear your mind of the day-to-day concerns so that you can brainstorm answers to the questions at hand. When I'm struggling with something, going into the silence almost always gives me the answer.

The best timing for this will vary from individual to individual. For morning people, it may be best to do this early in the morning, when you are fresh, and perhaps before the family gets up and the morning hustle begins. For night people, it may be best to do this late at night, after everyone else has retired. Or maybe just whenever you find a quiet moment.

How and where to work on developing your plan may also vary by individual. Going into the silence works especially well for introverts as they generally want to be by themselves anyway to think. They may even want to take a warm bath and sip a glass of wine before getting started. Some even do their best thinking on vacation while away from the normal routine. Extroverts, by contrast, may prefer to think out loud and be around others, and may be most energized by going to a party first. It's up to you. Just choose whatever works best for you to let you focus on these important, life-changing questions.

Brainstorm

The brainstorming part is pretty straightforward, but there are some rules. Just let whatever your brain hands you come out. Don't censor and don't evaluate at this point. Try to get as much of it out as fast as you can. Keep asking yourself the same question over and over—once the surface answers emerge, it's that deeper probing that produces the breakthrough answers.

Write It Down

Writing it down and getting it on paper would seem to be pretty obvious, but often is not. Writing it down is where the real power comes in. You're putting it into a tangible form so that you, and your subconscious mind, can work on it. Earlier I told you about how writing down my goal of a Dallas Business Journal column led to it actually happening—that's the power of writing it down.

For me, brainstorming and writing it down typically happens as a mind map, which is a very powerful visual tool. Mind maps start with a central concept in the middle of the page and develop as related ideas are drawn radiating outward. You draw pictures and connectors to show relationships—mind maps are powerful because they are pictorial. Feel free to do your plan with mind maps if that works well for you.

My goal throughout the rest of this book will be to give you tools and practical strategies, and to share my secrets, so that you can create a plan to save your own life.

During periods of relaxation after concentrated intellectual activity,
the intuitive mind seems to take over and can produce the sudden
clarifying insights which give so much joy and delight.
Fritjof Capra, Physicist and Author

Chapter

14

Where Do You Want To Go?

Before you can create your plan, you have to figure out what's important to you and where you want to go. As I mentioned, if you don't know where you want to go, any road will take you there.

In this chapter, we'll explore some basic questions, and then use them to put together your plan. This is the process that I used to figure out where I wanted to go—I'm sharing my story so that you can do better than I did. The questions are:

1) What are my values?

2) What are my actual and ideal priorities?

3) What would my ideal life look like?

4) How do I attain my ideal life?

5) When can I attain my ideal life?

Question 1: What Are My Values?

In exploring this first question, what are my values, think about the characteristics that you expect from yourself and value in others. This question is about the "what", not about the "how," which we'll deal with later.

Most of us tend to list values like honesty and integrity—those are often first on our lists. Other values tend to vary from one person's list to another. The sample below, in Figure 14.1, includes characteristics that I value.

My dad was the most principled person I've known, and he taught me his values, which is how honesty and integrity came to be what I value most.

Question 1: What Are My Values?

1.   Honesty
2.   Integrity
3.   Love
4.   Caring
5.   Understanding
6.   Self-reliance/independence
7.   Growth
8.   Health
9.   Passion for my mission/making a difference
10. Hard work
11. Teamwork/collaboration
12. Sharing

Figure 14.1: Sample Answers To Question 1, What Are My Values?

What do you value most? Fill out your own list of values, in Figure 14.2, either here or in the master list in Appendix A.

Question 1: What Are My Values?

1. _____
2. _____
3. _____
4. _____
5. _____
6. _____
7. _____
8. _____
9. _____
10. _____
11. _____
12. _____

Figure 14.2: Your Answers To Question 1, What Are My Values?

Question 2: What Are My Priorities?

This second question, what are my priorities, is about what is most important to you and will help you prioritize the components in your plan when you reach that step. In making a plan, sometimes people want to skip this part and move straight to the to-do list stage, but without knowing what is most important, how can they possibly know that once they accomplish their plan they will be fulfilled?

To answer this priorities question, think about what you value most. That will go under the column headed "Ideal." Your list might include family, career, health, religion or spiritual growth, social, and volunteerism. For simplicity sake, the sample in Figure 14.3 lists the usual top three priorities for most people—family, health, and job or career—in the Ideal column. I placed a number next to each priority in the Ideal column to indicate the order of importance.

Question 2: What Are My Ideal and Actual Priorities?	
Ideal	Actual
1. Family	1. Job/Career
2. Health	2. Family
3. Job/Career	3. Health

Figure 14.3: Sample Answers To Question 2, What Are My Ideal and Actual Priorities?

As we all know, life is a juggling act, so ideal priorities may not be the same as actual priorities, as exemplified by our lives. In real life, job or career frequently comes first due to job demands, and often squeezes out family and health. The sample above shows actual priorities that are different from the ideal ones.

I suspect that most of you can relate to that due to the pressures of today's work world and situations over which you don't have immediate control. Have you ever spent your anniversary, Valentine's Day, child's birthday, or your child's first day of school away from home simply because someone else chose to have a meeting then that you were expected or mandated to attend? I sure have. You may have felt that you couldn't influence it, or that requesting a change would be a career-limiting move. Or you just may have gotten shot down when you suggested a change. If so, then you understand the challenge of trying to stick to your priorities. If that's never happened to you, you've been mighty lucky, or were totally in control of your destiny.

I have a friend in a sales role that had to attend her company's annual sales meeting, a mandatory meeting for her job. It was halfway across the country, and she would be gone on the day that her son started first grade. It was so gut wrenching for her that after the first day of the sales meeting, she packed up and headed home so she could be there for his first day of school. She knew what her priorities were and acted upon them.

Prior to my heart incident, family was my top priority, job was second, and health was third. Sometimes, however, because I was on the road a lot, my job got in the way of family and health.

In some industries, high tech for one, the productivity treadmill constantly speeds up, with job demands seemingly increasing exponentially. As a result of these work pressures, my job seemed to absorb every available minute, taking my evenings, especially on the road, and a lot of my weekends for projects and expectations that just couldn't get done during the week. The time for focusing on my health just seemed to evaporate.

Many of us women don't put enough emphasis on our health, until it is too late. Remember that oxygen mask.

Now, in Figure 14.4, fill in your own ideal and actual priorities, in the order of their priority.

Question 2: What Are My Ideal and Actual Priorities?	
Ideal	Actual
1. _____	1. _____
2. _____	2. _____
3. _____	3. _____
4. _____	4. _____
5. _____	5. _____
6. _____	6. _____
7. _____	7. _____

Figure 14.4: Your Answers to Question 2, What Are My Ideal and Actual Priorities?

Does your actual match your ideal? Are you walking your talk? Most likely not, and it may not be your fault. It's a reality in today's world, especially if you travel a lot, or are in a field or geographic area where there is a lot of job insecurity. Many of you may be in areas, such as IT, call center, or engineering, where offshore outsourcing is obliterating jobs. When there are no jobs to transition to, we are often forced to do things that we would prefer not to, such as working long hours, not standing up for our personal lives, or not taking vacation for fear of coming back to no job.

My family is most important to me. Having this life-changing experience altered what I must do to be there for them. The challenge for me, as I faced my mortality, was not only how to continue to be there for them, but also how to avoid having more surgery. I knew I had to make changes in how I implemented my priorities.

Question 3: What Would My Ideal Life Look Like?

The third question, what would my ideal life look like, is perfect for going into the silence to visualize and let your inner thoughts emerge. Explore your dreams, hopes, vision, mission, and goals. Probe your innermost thoughts for what success does, and should, look like for you. Think about how you will know if you're successful.

As I probed these kinds of questions after my surgery, I thought about what I wanted to accomplish, and in what time frame. As I mentioned earlier, I felt there was something that I was supposed to do with my second chance, but wasn't quite sure what it was or how to go about it.

I mentioned earlier that just three weeks after surgery I had shared my experience and what women need to know about heart disease with almost one hundred women at Leadership Texas. As I reconnected with these friends, I realized how passionate I was about helping others. As I shared what I had learned, I was touched by their responses. The final morning of Leadership Texas, we did an exercise to explore what we truly wanted to do and here's what I wrote down for my ideal life:

- Touch people's lives through my experience and story

- Have a healthy family, and travel with them around the country in the motorhome, speaking about health and wellness

- Be a healthy, successful speaker and writer (success meant changing lives, not being rich or famous)

When I came home I developed a plan, boiling the list down to the three goals shown in Figure 14.5, below.

Question 3: What Would My Ideal Life Look Like?
1. Be healthy and well to save my own life 2. Have a healthy family 3. Make a difference in peoples' lives

Figure 14.5: Sample Answers to Question 3, What Would My Ideal Life Look Like?

My Leadership Texas experience helped me start realizing my passion to make a difference in women's lives. My story could be a cautionary tale of what not to do, and I could provide information that others might not know. After all, they could still prevent heart disease, even if I could not.

Did I go home and quit my job right away? Of course not. However, I started thinking through how I might do this, starting with getting myself healthy and focusing on my family. Then I would pursue my mission, turning it into my life's work and career.

When I started getting my health under control, and found that volunteering as a speaker for the American Heart Association was fulfilling, I continued the soul searching. On my trip to Italy, discussions with my mother and sisters helped me make the final decision to pursue this mission full-time.

What do you want to accomplish? What would your ideal life look like? In Figure 14.6, brainstorm and fill in your answers.

Question 3: What Would My Ideal Life Look Like?
1. _____ 2. _____ 3. _____ 4. _____ 5. _____ 6. _____ 7. _____

Figure 14.6: Your Answers to Question 3, What Would My Ideal Life Look Like?

Once you've decided, should you keep this as a secret or should you share it with others? That depends on your environment. Are the people with whom you would share it supportive? Are they willing to help you accomplish your goals? If so, then by all means share this so they can start helping you accomplish your dreams. If people around you are negative naysayers who may tear down your dreams, then keep it to yourself. If they are toxic and negative, you just may have to consider backing away from them. Figure out who can support you in building your dreams, and look to them for support and help.

Question 4: How Do I Attain My Ideal Life?

For the fourth question, how do I attain my ideal life, use your list from Figure 14.6 and break it down into the next level of detail. We'll look at where you want to go, where you are now, and how to bridge that gap.

In the sample, in Figure 14.7, I broke out the components of my first goal, Be Healthy and Well. Those components, in the Ideal column, included to reach my optimal weight, have excellent cholesterol and blood pressure, be energetic, be relaxed and in control, be rested and rejuvenated, be more proactive with my health, and to have a balanced life.

Question 4: How Do I Attain My Ideal Life?
1. Be Healthy and Well

Actual	Ideal	How to Bridge the Gap
Overweight	Optimal weight	Restore normal weight through diet and exercise
Good cholesterol and blood pressure	Excellent cholesterol and blood pressure	Maintain and monitor
Tired	Energetic	Build energy and stamina through exercise
Overstressed and overloaded	Relaxed and in control	Decrease stress through taking control
Sleep-deprived and mentally fatigued	Rested and rejuvenated	Get rest and relaxation
Proactive with health	More proactive with health	Lots of research and study
Stretched too thinly	Balanced life	Outside interests

Figure 14.7: Sample Answers to Question 4, How Do I Attain My Ideal Life?

I then identified where I was at the time and what I needed to do to bridge the gap. For example, at the time (just after my surgery) I was overweight and needed to restore my normal weight through diet and exercise.

One major input in creating this list was the list of risk factors from my own risk assessment, like the one in Figure 7.9. I was at risk in numbers 6 (overweight), 7 (activity), and 8 (stress). I also realized that it was important to keep my vital statistics under control, so even though numbers 3 (blood pressure) and 4 (cholesterol) were under control, I wanted to be vigilant in maintaining and monitoring them.

Now it's now your turn. In Figure 14.8, fill in your own answers about how to attain your ideal life. Since you probably bought this book to improve your health or avoid illness, the risk factors you listed in your risk assessment in Figure 7.9 should be a basis for some of your answers. For example, if you smoke, you might add being smoke-free under the ideal column. Once you have filled in the ideal, then back up to identify where you are now (actual) and how to bridge the gap between your actual and ideal.

Question 4: How Do I Attain My Ideal Life?

Actual	Ideal	How to Bridge the Gap

Figure 14.8: Your Answers to Question 4, How Do I Attain My Ideal Life?

Question 5: When Can I Attain My Ideal Life?

In the fifth question, when can I attain my ideal life, use the steps you created to bridge the gap in Figure 14.8, above, and identify the dates by which you plan to accomplish them.

Question 5: When Can I Attain My Ideal Life?

Goals / Objectives	Completion Date
1. Be healthy & well to save my life	
Restore normal weight (lose XX pounds)—fat-free diet now	12 months
Build stamina & energy from exercising 30–60 minutes/day	1 month
Decrease stress by taking back control	1 month
Get rest—7–8 hours sleep per night	1 month
Get relaxation—plan & take motorhome vacation with family	2 months
Take proactive control of health through research	1 month
Maintain good blood pressure & cholesterol, & increase HDL	1 month
Engage in outside interests	2 months
2. Make a difference in people's lives	
Develop business plan for making a living	3 months
Speak on health/preventing heart disease	
Volunteer for American Heart Association	2 months
Research and create speech	2 months
Deliver first AHA speech	3 months
Travel in motorhome w/ family to speak	6 months
Write about health/preventing disease	6 months

Figure 14.9: Sample Answers to Question 5, When Can I Attain My Ideal Life?

In the sample plan in Figure 14.9, you see two of my goals, Be Healthy and Well and Make a Difference in People's Lives, broken down into detailed steps, with target completion dates listed for each.

The challenge in setting a plan is often in determining the dates by which you will reach your goals. There are two ways to figure this out.

1)   List the steps, and the time that each will take, and use that to set your expected completion date, or

2)   Decide when you'd like to have accomplished your ideal life, and work backward to fill in the dates.

For example, in my sample plan in Figure 14.9, I set the date for "get relaxation—plan and take motorhome vacation with family" for two months out, and then worked backwards with the details to make it happen then. Use the approach that suits you best.

In setting all the dates, I took into consideration that I still had a full-time road warrior job requiring lots of hours and travel. Otherwise, I could have done these much faster. Of course, this is only a sample plan.

Most of us overestimate how soon we can accomplish individual steps, so don't flog yourself if you don't make it by then. We also underestimate what we can actually accomplish in a lifetime, so don't cheat yourself by not stretching far enough. It may be better to aim high rather than to aim too low, but give yourself permission to reach your goal through a series of intermediate goals if that works best for you. We women know how to accomplish goals; we just need to make sure that we focus those goals on us, rather than on our jobs.

Let me reemphasize the power of writing this down. On January 1, a few months after leaving my road warrior job, I updated my plan and added new personal and business goals. One goal was to raise women's awareness about heart disease by appearing on local TV by the end of June, and on national TV by the end of the year. Amazingly the next day I got a flood of e-mails from friends saying that some friends who produce for PBS were doing a show about heart disease. I shared my story with the host, and he booked me to appear. The show aired in Dallas and in cities around the country. Then in February, I spoke at the local press conference kicking off the American Heart Association's "Go Red for Women" program to raise women's awareness of heart disease. Interviews appeared on three local TV stations that evening and my story appeared in the newspaper. Does writing it down work? You bet it does.

In Figure 14.10, fill in your steps and dates to reach your ideal life. It's fine to have interim goals, with multiple steps and dates, as I did in number two in the sample where I put in multiple steps for reaching my goal of speaking about health.

I used time frames in my sample to make it more relevant when you read this, but in your case put in actual dates so that you can feel ownership for, and excitement about, your plan.

Consider how much time you can realistically devote to it. If it requires a job change, how much time will that take, especially if the economy or job outlook still isn't very robust? It won't happen overnight, so don't expect it. If it does, you'll be pleasantly surprised. You know that you can do whatever you set you mind to.

Question 5: When Can I Attain My Ideal Life?	
Goals / Objectives	Completion Date

Figure 14.10: Your Answers to Question 5, When Can I Attain My Ideal Life?

We've just finished exploring where you want to go. I'm going to presume that the reason you chose this book was because you want to improve your health and to live longer, so for the rest of the book we will focus on practical strategies for fulfilling your health goals. Chapter 15 provides the foundation for creating your own HEART Program. The plan you created in Figure 14.10 will be the basis from which to develop your HEART Program.

You must be the change you wish to see in the world.
Mahatma Gandhi, 1869–1948, Indian Political Leader

Chapter
15

Creating Your HEART Program

The HEART Program is what I created to take control of my health and to avoid future heart and other health issues. It consists of the following components, which we will explore in great detail in Chapters 16–20:

H: Healthy Eating: How I Lost 85 Pounds and You Can Lose, Too

E: Exercise Daily

A: Attitude Toward Stress: How You Can Learn to Love Stress

R: Rest, Relaxation, and Rejuvenation

T: Take Proactive Control of Your Health

Sample HEART Program Action Plan

The HEART Program Action Plan that we will create in this chapter brings together two items that you have already created:

1) Your Risk Assessment from Figure 7.9

2) Your Ideal Life Goals and Completion Dates from Figure 14.10

Let's look at how that will come together by using the sample in Figure 15.1, below.

This sample (these are not my numbers) was created from a risk assessment done using the same form that you used in Figure 7.9. To create this sample, I transferred the contents of the "Risk Y/N" column on the risk assessment to the Risk column here. For those with a risk (Y), or those that I wished to focus on, I transferred the readings in the Current column (blood pressure, cholesterol, etc.) there to the Current column here. I used the numbers in the Normal/Ideal column there to determine what to use in the Ideal/Goal column here.

**HEART Program
Action Plan**

Risk Factor/ Measures	Risk	Current	Ideal/ Goal	Gap	Action/ Step(s)	Target Date
1. Smoking	N					
2. Diabetes Blood glucose	N					
3. Blood pressure	N	106/94			Maintain	
4. Cholesterol	Y				Fat-free diet	1 mo
Total		210	<200	≥10↓	Statin	1 mo
Triglycerides		155	<150	≥ 5↓	Research	1 mo
LDL (Bad)		135	<130	≥ 5↓		
HDL (Good)		35	>50	≥15↑	Exercise 30m	1 mo
5. Family history	N					
6. Overweight	Y					
Height						
Weight (1st goal)		160	150	10	Low-fat diet	3 mo
BMI						
Waist						
Weight class						
Risk (BMI/waist)						
Weight (2nd goal)		150	140	10	Low-fat diet	6 mo
7. Activity level	Y	Low	Medium	Small	Exercise 30m	1 mo
8. Stress	Y	High	Low	Large	Take control	1 mo
					Sleep 8 hrs	1 mo
					Relax/vacation	2 mo
					Activities	2 mo
9. Other	_					

Figure 15.1: Sample HEART Program Action Plan

For purposes of the sample, these items were risks or concerns:

1) Cholesterol (4) – risk

2) Overweight (6) – risk

3) Activity level (7) – risk

4) Stress (8) – risk

5) Blood pressure (3) – concern

In addition to the four risks, cholesterol, overweight, activity level, and stress, we are focusing on one area that isn't a risk, blood pressure, so that we keep it from becoming a risk.

By using the current and ideal numbers in the sample I calculated the gaps to address and started listing the action steps and target dates for addressing those gaps.

Some of the action steps were identified by doing a sample version like what you did in Figure 14.10, and a few were pulled from the sample I used in Figure 14.9. Some action steps, such as getting the cholesterol numbers down, involve multiple steps—in this case the multiple steps include a fat-free diet, a statin drug, exercise to increase the good cholesterol, and research to understand how to get and keep cholesterol under control. There are many things to know about the impact of different foods on cholesterol levels, so you will find a lot of guidance about that in the next chapter.

Since activity level (7) and stress (8) can't be easily quantified in numbers, I used descriptions there to indicate current, ideal, and gap.

There are multiple lines for each category since sometimes the best results come from having interim goals. It can be hard to make a big jump all at once, so interim goals are much easier to reach, and are less frustrating. In the sample, the first weight goal in the overweight category was to get from a current weight of 160 pounds (just an example) to a goal of 150 pounds, a gap of 10 pounds, shown as a 3 month goal. On the next blank line, which is at the bottom of the overweight category, is the second weight goal, to get from a then-current weight of 150 pounds to a goal of 140, another 10 pound gap, shown as an additional 3 months, for a target completion date in 6 months.

Having interim goals is a mind trick—a ten pound goal is infinitely easier than a twenty pound goal, and when you show current weight of 150 for the second goal, the brain sees the first goal as having been reached, sending a very powerful message to your subconscious mind.

Your HEART Program Action Plan

Now fill out Figure 15.2 with your action plan. Start by transferring your risks and current measures from Figure 7.9, and use the normal/ideal measures there to decide on what your goals should be. Then calculate the gap and use your plan in Figure 14.10 to develop your own action steps and target dates, like what you saw in the sample. Where I used time frames in the sample so it would make sense when you read this, it should be easier for you to use actual dates. Just in case you have other relevant measures that you keep tabs on, I left blanks for that in number 9 at the bottom.

As you fill this out, please keep in mind that ideal weight doesn't mean someone else's idea of what your weight should be—it's what you believe is a healthy weight for you. That's not necessarily what your doctor says or what the standard weight tables say. Most of us know the weight at which we are healthiest. Notice that I said healthy, not skinny.

Looking like a supermodel is not what we're after here. (After the age of 25, they can't keep looking like that either!) We're looking for good health.

Risk Factor/ Measures	Risk	Current	Ideal/ Goal	Gap	Action/ Step(s)	Target Date
HEART Program Action Plan						
1. Smoking	—					
2. Diabetes Blood glucose	—					
3. Blood pressure	—					
4. Cholesterol Total Triglycerides LDL (Bad) HDL (Good)	—					
5. Family history	—					
6. Overweight Height Weight (1st goal) BMI Waist Weight class Risk (BMI/waist) Weight (2nd goal)	—					
7. Activity level	—					
8. Stress	—					
9. Other	—					

Figure 15.2: Your HEART Program Action Plan

Now that you know the details of what you want to address, we'll delve into the "how." Over the next five chapters, we'll explore the details of the HEART Program for taking care of your heart and your health. The individual steps, shown below, are tied to the individual risk factors focused on in Figure 15.2, above.

H: Healthy Eating: How I Lost 85 Pounds And You Can Lose, Too (Chapter 16)

E: Exercise Daily (Chapter 17)

A: Attitude Toward Stress: How You Can Learn to Love Stress (Chapter 18)

R: Rest, Relaxation, and Rejuvenation (Chapter 19)

T: Take Proactive Control of Your Health (Chapter 20)

Finally, in Chapter 21 we will wrap it all up with Putting It All Together and Making a Commitment.

Getting my lifelong weight struggle under control has come from a process of treating myself as well as I treat others.
Oprah Winfrey, 1954– , Actress and TV talk show host

Chapter

16

Healthy Eating: How I Lost 85 Pounds and You Can Lose, Too

In this chapter, we'll focus on what keeps us from eating a healthy diet, what are the options if we need to lose weight, what are the pros and cons regarding certain popular diets, what is the most heart-healthy way to eat, and how to plan for your own healthy eating. By the end of this chapter you will have evaluated your choices and have put together a plan customized for you.

The Problems of Our Twenty-first Century Diets

With the time pressures impacting us today, it is really hard to eat healthfully. Do you ever find that there's just too much to do to find time for healthy eating? With work, family, and more and more activities shoehorned into every day, how do we find the time? We often don't.

Do you run family and personal errands at lunch, maybe eating a fast food lunch, or even worse, eating from the vending machine? Or do you work through lunch? With the increased work demands that we all face, and the increased need to multitask, a recent CNBC poll found that 67% of us eat lunch at our desks.

What about after work? Do you run a carload of kids to baseball or soccer, grabbing "drive-by" food enroute? When they were babies, and you had to choose between eating and showering that day, did you realize that you were practicing to be a soccer mom? It can get so crazy running from work to family activities that rush hour traffic sometimes feels like the calm between the storms?

We're now a "fast-food" nation, and though we know it's not the healthiest way to eat, what can we do? Fast food makes juggling the day-to-day demands easier, but it also helps pile on the pounds, and is largely responsible for so many Americans being overweight.

When former president Bill Clinton had heart bypass surgery, the media kept showing photos of Clinton in McDonalds, a reference to his penchant for fast food. And in the recent movie, "Super-Size Me", the main character did an experiment by eating every meal at McDonalds, super-sizing when asked, and finishing whatever he was served. Not only did he pile on the pounds, but also increased his cholesterol to the point where his doctor begged him to call off the experiment due to the risk to his health.

Do you ever eat to feel better? Is that a frequent occurrence? It easily can be when you have major stressors in your life. When you're under stress on the job, or from caring for aging parents, it's amazing what chocolate can do!

For me, my eating challenge was being on the road constantly, and having marathon meetings, with no time to grab food, much less healthy food. Changing time zones didn't help either. After September 11, in-flight meals went away, at least on the flights I was on. Carrying food through security checkpoints was asking for trouble, but it was no better trying to find healthy food in airports. Fortunately, some airport fast-food shops do have to-go salads, maybe even with grilled chicken. Adding a low-fat or fat-free dressing, even if it meant carrying my own packages, usually worked, and if all else failed, I could squeeze on lemon or sprinkle on vinegar to substitute for dressing.

Bottom line: Our crazy diets are a product of our crazy lives.

Which Diet Is Best For You?

As you've read, being overweight puts us at increased risk for heart disease and heart attack. Losing excess weight decreases the risk. In Chapter 15, you identified whether you need to lose weight and/or modify your eating to bring your cholesterol or blood glucose under control. In this section, we will help you choose the right diet for doing that.

Roughly two-thirds of Americans are overweight, and since many of us women are perpetually on diets, sometimes moving from one to another like we change outfits, it's good to know that losing weight (not to excess) is heart-friendly. Even if you're not overweight, a heart-smart diet is necessary for keeping cholesterol and blood pressure under control.

Before my heart surgery, I was overweight, though I had already lost twenty-two pounds. I knew I needed to lose even more, but my cardiologist gave me a nudge. OK, so maybe it was more like a 2x4 over the head. Whatever! He arranged for the hospital nutritionist to visit to give me information about how to eat to lose weight so I wouldn't end up back in the hospital.

I thought I already knew a lot about nutrition from college, having taken nutrition courses along with the required chemistry (organic, inorganic, biochemistry—the works) and physics. I tolerated nutrition, but thought it was very boring. Looking back, it's probably one of the things that helped save my life. And it sure made it easier to delve back into nutrition for my own health. From the hospital nutritionist, I learned that much has changed in the nutrition field.

In helping you with your diet, I could recommend that each of you go out and get a thick new college textbook on nutrition and read it, but most of you would be asleep before you finished page 2. To avoid that, in this chapter I'll boil down what you need to know and concentrate on the major things that are important for your overall health.

How do you choose the right diet from all the possible options? Should you go low-carb, the latest blockbuster diet rage? The Atkins and South Beach diets seem to have taken over the world. Or should you go with a traditional low-fat diet? What about The Zone or Ornish? Which diet is best? How do you choose? The American Heart Association recently studied the effectiveness of four very popular diets—Atkins, the Zone, Ornish, and traditional low-fat—and found that all yielded about a 5% average weight loss coupled with a 7–15% reduction in heart disease risk. Losing just a few pounds reduces the risk of heart disease, and since they all work, it's your choice.

In choosing a diet, however, remember that balance is a good thing. Nutritionists caution that staying on a diet long term that eliminates a major nutrition item, such as carbs or fats, is a bad thing. According to one physician, staying on Atkins long-term can lead to kidney damage, but for short-term use it appears to be OK, and is often correlated with decreased cholesterol levels that are heart-healthy. Maybe I should also clarify here that my version of a fat-free diet avoids or minimizes the bad fats, but I do eat the good ones. Perhaps I should call it a "*bad-fat* free diet"—that's too complicated, so when I mention fat-free, please think of it in those terms.

Defying conventional wisdom, two recent research studies showed that low-carb diets result in more weight loss over the first six months than do low-fat diets, though after twelve months the losses equalize. Being overweight is a significant health risk, and either diet will reduce your overall risk.

A couple of caveats: Participants in both studies ate mostly meats and vegetables, with very little processed food, so having a diet high in convenience foods may yield very different results. All the new low-carb products, from companies such as Coca-Cola and Nestlé, haven't been factored into the low-carb studies yet. In addition, low-fat dieters limited themselves to 30% or fewer calories from fats, which could be slightly on the high side for dieting and may explain the slower weight loss.

In the studies, low-carb dieters also reaped heart-healthy benefits from lowered triglyceride levels and higher levels of good (HDL) cholesterol. However, the impact on the bad (LDL) cholesterol was scary—low-carb dieters saw increased LDL levels of up to 10%, while low-fat dieters saw decreases.

Recent research indicates that you should get your LDL as low as it will go to lessen your heart disease risk. Because of the impact on LDL, if you have heart risk factors, such as high cholesterol or high blood pressure, you should only pursue a low-carb diet under doctor's supervision. In the meantime, the Atkins diet is being revised to recommend limiting consumption of meat, cheese, and dairy, making it lower in fat, potentially decreasing the impact on LDL.

In spite of good short-term results from low-carb diets, doctors continue to express reservations about the long-term impact of low-carb diets since insufficient intake of fiber and nutrients correlates with heart disease, cancer, and kidney problems.

For some strange reason, I'm always going against the grain (no pun intended). For decades, I tended toward a low-carb diet by not eating breads or cereals, though I did get fiber from veggies. Breads and cereals seemed like such a waste of perfectly good calories, and since I limited my daily calories, I preferred to apply them elsewhere.

Now that I have heart disease, I've had to add back lots of grains to my new fat-free diet, just as the rest of the world has gone low carb. The hospital nutritionist insisted that I add breads and other fiber to my diet, concentrating on more servings of fiber than anything else. I already had lots of fiber from fruits and veggies, but I've had to add grains to my diet, too.

Did all those years of bunless burgers and breadless sandwiches have anything to do with my heart disease? Based on what doctors and nutritionists are saying about lack of fiber in low-carb diets putting you at risk of heart disease, it just possibly could be related.

With the addition of fiber to my diet, I occasionally now even eat foods that I grew up thinking of as being fattening. I had typically avoided corn as my grandmother used to say, "You can't reduce a corn-fed gal!" Did you hear that growing up, too? Well, maybe that was only those of us who grew up in the South. But corn contains fiber, which is now a necessity. Since I'm on a blood-thinner that requires consistent intake of Vitamin K (found in green foods), I've had to closely regulate my broccoli and salad green consumption, which is frustrating as they are low in calories and are good for you. That's a problem since I'm allergic to legumes and have had to find other veggies to rely on. Now that the world has moved from low fat to low carb, I'm totally out of sync.

What is the best diet? Low-carb diets seem to be working great for a large percentage of the population (at least in the US). I know many people, including family members, who have experienced dramatic weight loss on Atkins. From what I'd heard and read in the media, I thought we were all on low-carb diets—except for me, that is. That doesn't appear to be the case. A recent survey that I conducted provided some surprising results. Perhaps individual doctors are warning patients about the health impact of low-carb diets, or perhaps low-carb diets don't work for everyone.

The survey was unscientific, and the sample size was small, but it does indicate a potential trend. I surveyed readers of my Healthy Living News e-zine as well as those on an all-female distribution list that I maintain. I also factored in responses to my questions posed on the discussion forum of WITI (Women in Technology International, http://www.witi.com). Therefore, a high percentage of the responses came from women.

I asked what kind of diet readers were on (low carb, low fat, other, or none), and their experiences with them, including the effect on health measures such as cholesterol and blood pressure. The chart below, in Figure 16.1, shows the diet survey results.

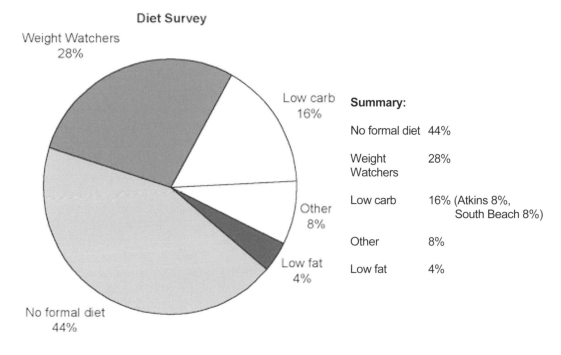

Figure 16.1: Diet Survey Results

While I fully expected that almost no one would be on a low-fat diet, I was stunned that nearly half (44%) weren't on any diet at all. Some women's magazines reinforce the myth that all women are on diets, which obviously isn't so. However, as many discussed their own approaches to healthy eating, including smaller portions, more fruits and vegetables, and eating less meat and dairy, many of them sounded very similar to a low fat diet.

It was surprising that only 8% were on Atkins and 8% were on South Beach. The first hint that I had about waning low-carb popularity came in talking with a friend who owns some restaurants. She mentioned that her low-carb sales had started out well, but have languished recently. The survey seems to have corroborated that.

Most surprising was the 28% on Weight Watchers, many of whom had abandoned diets such as Atkins and South Beach and were now happily maintaining their weight with Weight Watchers. Several referred to it as a Life Plan for eating, not a diet.

In Figure 16.2, you'll find a flavor of what I heard regarding diets and eating plans, as well as their results. These are summaries to give you a feel for the trends, not exact quotes.

Diet Survey Comments

Atkins (Low-carb):

❑ Low-fat didn't work for me in running marathons, as I had no endurance and stamina. I did low carb on my doctor's recommendation. Now, I not only have endurance for marathons, but my cholesterol and blood pressure are also the lowest ever.

❑ I lost 48 pounds on Atkins and have maintained it. In addition, my cholesterol and blood pressure are down.

South Beach (Low-carb):

❑ It works for me because it's both low-fat and low-carb. I get more fruits and vegetables than Atkins.

❑ It's healthy because it focuses on minimal saturated fat and processed foods, and lets you have lots of low-fat foods and moderate amounts of whole grains.

Weight Watchers:

❑ WW is a Life Plan. I've been on it for 3 1/2 yrs and have lost 50+ pounds. I can make choices of what to eat. I usually eat fruits and vegetables with a small portion of meat. If I want a glass of wine, I can have it.

❑ On Atkins, I lost 18 pounds in 2 months, but I dreaded meals as I prefer veggies to meat. When I stopped Atkins, I regained all the weight in 1 month. Now, with WW, I have reached my goal and have maintained it. I'm in control and know how to manage my weight.

❑ I lost 21 pounds on Weight Watchers. This is the first time I've chosen to stop losing rather than hitting a plateau that I couldn't break through. I choose to eat low fat as I can get more food. My cholesterol and glucose are both down as a result.

Diet Survey Comments

❑   I use the online Weight Watchers—it's easy and less expensive than the meetings.

No formal plan:

❑   South Beach was difficult to stay on, so I just eat breakfast, and have a smaller lunch and dinner.

❑   I lost 80 pounds from eating smaller portions of a balanced diet, and getting lots of exercise. I've kept it off for over a year.

❑   I simply cut back on quantities when the scale starts going up.

❑   I avoid diets and scales, sticking to a balance of healthy foods and exercise.

❑   I don't do diets—I follow the USDA food pyramid.

Other:

❑   "How Sugar Makes Us Crazy, Sick, & Fat" by Joan Ifland.

❑   "The Detox Diet" by Dr. Paula Baillie-Hamilton (through Shaklee).

❑   Gastric bypass—it's wonderful.

Low-fat:

❑   I stick to low fat (minimal meat and dairy) with lots of fruits, veggies, and some whole grains.

Figure 16.2: Diet Survey Comments

When contemplating diets or new eating plans, I think it's often helpful to learn from the experiences of other women, and to hear their experiences in their own words. Here, in Figure 16.3, are some quotes from those who have been there, and what they found worked best for them.

Women's Diet Experiences

I've been on low-carb, via Atkins, for about 2 years. It was originally recommended by my doctor to help me lower my cholesterol/blood pressure. It has worked wonderfully, and today's blood pressure at 129/72 was the lowest it's been in years and years! My total cholesterol is under 200 for the first time in my adult life!

Additionally, an unexpected reaction is this: I find as an athlete that I'm much, much stronger and my endurance is clearly better than ever before. My reading tells me that because I was eating so low-fat/high-carb before that when I was doing 3 or 4 hours of running or triathlons, I was bonking because I couldn't eat enough to keep up! Now that my body is "trained" to burn fat I feel much better on the long runs (over 90 minutes, etc.)

--Susan Baughman, Professional speaker

Women's Diet Experiences

I just had to let you know that my change in eating and exercise habits has paid off—the proof is in the blood tests. Over the last year and a half, while on the South Beach plan, I have cut my triglycerides in half, raised my good cholesterol, and lowered my bad cholesterol, so my risk ratio is 1.08—an all-time record low for me.

I have also been able, under a doctor's supervision, to curtail my blood pressure medicine and other medications.

Combine that with 3–5 hours of exercise a week and I now hope to live to be 100!!

--Carla Daws, Texas state government agency

I'm on the South Beach Diet. I lost 12 pounds last September and, to date, have kept it off with a maintenance program. The year before that I lost 10 pounds due to a ton of exercise in preparation for an event. The training did not stay at the same pace so I had to look for an eating program.

My plan was to lose 10 or so pounds and keep it off for a year. The following year I would lose another 10 pounds, etc. This September, I'll try to lose my last 10 pounds to reach my goal. It's slow, but my body and appetite need the time to get used to the weight.

South Beach appealed to me because of its lo-fat/lo-carb approach. There are more vegetables on the plan, and you can have fruit after the first two weeks. Plus, it's a cheatable diet. I was on Weight Watchers prior to South Beach and found that I was eating all carbs to keep my points low, and therefore was hungry all the time. Having less sugar in my system keeps my cravings down.

--Vicki, Austin, TX

I guess technically South Beach is low-carb, but I think that is just marketing hype. In reality, it's the way we should all be eating—a minimum of saturated fats, minimum of processed foods (especially sugar), and lots of low-fat foods and a moderate amount of healthy whole grains.

--Karen Hiser, www.HealthyTravelNetwork.com

I diligently followed the Atkins diet for 2+ months and was successful in dropping most of my unwanted weight (about 18 lbs out of a goal of 23 lbs), however, I got to the point where I almost dreaded meal times since I'm much more of a veggie person than a meat eater. That finally got to me and I went off the diet. What followed is what really blew me away...within 1 month I had gained back every pound that I lost over 2+ months. I've NEVER gained weight that fast in my life.

I decided I had to take a different route. So, in late September, 2003, I joined Weight Watchers. By Thanksgiving, I had reached my goal weight. By January, I had maintained my weight at or below goal long enough to achieve Lifetime Membership status. I have remained at or below my goal weight ever since and am still actively attending meetings at least once per month. The balance and choice that the Weight Watchers program provides really makes me feel like I'm in control and know how to manage my weight. It's been great and I haven't felt at all deprived.

--Karlene Seime-Noble, Financial industry executive

Women's Diet Experiences

I have been on Weight Watchers Life Plan for over 3 1/2 years. (They don't call it a diet.) I lost a total of 50 lbs and have kept it off for 3 years.

Weight Watchers is neither low fat nor low carb—we practice portion control and eat from all food groups in a healthy manner. In Weight Watchers you are empowered to make choices so if I want my glass of wine for dinner, I do so, count the points, and don't have dessert!

When I travel and attend conferences where the meals are rich, I eat a small portion of the entree, the salad, a half a roll, and three bites of dessert, and I am good to go! I eat lots of fruits and vegetables and 3–4 ounces of meat at dinner and sometimes at lunch.

--Cheri Butler, cbutlerlpc@yahoo.com

In 1999, I joined a study by Fred Hutchinson Cancer Research and the University of Washington to see if a diet low in fat and high in fruits and vegetables would help an esophagus condition developed as a result of acid reflux. We had to keep a food diary and count fat grams and fruit and vegetable servings (no calorie counting). I reduced my fat intake from around 52 grams a day to an average of 24, and ate anywhere from 6 to 10 or more servings of fruits and vegetables. I also cut down a bit on the quantity of starchy foods I ate.

I am 5 feet tall and weighed 143 lb. at the start of the program. I dropped about 12 lb, and then hit a plateau. I got an Internet-enabled treadmill and began downloading a daily 30-minute workout four or five times a week, plus on weekends I would take long walks (3–4 mi). Over a year I got down to 115, for a total loss of 28 lb.

When the study ended, my weight began creeping up again. In late summer 2003, I joined Weight Watchers and weighed in at 124.5. I reached my 115-lb goal weight in 4 months, but during the 6-week maintenance period, I continued to lose. Even after I became a Lifetime Member, I continued to lose until I got down to 103, which is pretty close to the minimum weight for my height, so I stopped. I do think this is a program that will help me keep the weight off for life, and I'm very glad to have found it!

--Carol, Bellevue, Washington

I tried the South Beach and did see some weight loss. I have a difficult time staying on diets. I try to always have breakfast and small lunches and dinners. I have not gone up significantly in weight from one year to the next. My nurse practitioner was happy with that but put me on a statin drug because she felt that I was borderline on my blood pressure. It has given me more energy and I am now able to increase my exercising without as much fatigue.

--Norma Almanza, Texas state government agency

I am not now, nor have I ever been, on one of those diets. I do not believe in any of them. I am a firm believer in following the USDA food pyramid and incorporating exercise into your life.

--Martha Alikacem, Insurance industry executive

Figure 16.3: Women's Diet Experiences

It's obvious that diets are so individual that you have to experiment to find what works best for you. You also have to stay up on the latest health research to make sure new findings don't call into question what your diet does for your health.

Recently there has been more bad news for low-carb dieters. It appears that low-carb diets make it harder for women to get pregnant. There are some segments of the population for whom this is good news—I understand that Atkins is very popular on campus. But, for others, this new information could be a serious setback and could cause a migration away from low-carb diets.

Now, a group called the Partnership for Essential Nutrition (http://www.essentialnutrition.org) is rallying to educate consumers about the value of healthy carbohydrates. This isn't some scheme by farmers or food manufacturers to discredit low-carb diets—founding coalition members include the American Association of Diabetes Educators, the American Institute for Cancer Research, the American Obesity Association, the National Women's Health Resource Center, the University of California at Davis Department of Nutrition, and others.

The coalition's concerns center around what low-carb diets are doing to American eating habits. Their goal is to raise awareness of the importance of carbohydrates in the diet for fueling the brain and the muscles. In addition, studies have proven that carbohydrates help to control weight and to lower the risk for stroke, heart disease, high blood pressure, and some cancers.

Many who are not on low-carb diets have the perception that carbs are unhealthy and have therefore decreased their overall consumption of fruits, vegetables, and grains—a very unhealthy trend. Fortunately, many consumers are now getting the message that carbs, in moderation, are actually good for you. As a result, according to market research firm Opinion Dynamics, the number who restrict their carbs but aren't on a low-carb diet decreased from 32 per cent in April, 2004 to 21 per cent in July, 2004, a very significant drop.

If you're considering a low-carb diet, it may be worth the time to check out the information on the Essential Nutrition site.

We may see a diet boomerang among Boomers. Where many are on low-carb diets today, health problems may cause them to swing back to low-fat eating. While Bill Clinton was on the South Beach diet before his heart bypass, it's very likely that his doctors put him on a low-fat diet afterwards.

Recommendation: Saving your own life is about healthy eating for a lifetime. While low-carb diets take off weight quickly and were way ahead of low-fat diets at the six month mark, after twelve months the weight loss was equal. You may want to do a diet of some kind to take off the weight rapidly and then consider switching to a reduced-fat healthy eating plan, as described in the next section. It is not only heart-healthy, but it also includes many of the nutritional elements needed to avoid cancer. This is the plan to follow for a lifetime of good health.

Plan for a Lifetime of Healthy Eating

The guidelines for healthy eating discussed in this section were recommended by my cardiologist and the hospital nutritionist, and are based on the recommendations of the American Heart Association (AHA) for a lifetime of healthy eating.

The AHA recommends that you eat fruits and vegetables, fish, poultry, limited lean meats, and lots of grains. The grains might include flaxseed and certain nuts to boost the Omega-3 fatty acids in your diet. The AHA suggests avoiding trans fat and saturated fat through minimizing dairy, or consuming fat-free dairy products, and significantly decreasing your consumption of fat-laden fast foods and baked goods.

The AHA Food Pyramid (http://www.deliciousdecisions.org/ee/afp.html) is adapted from the US Department of Agriculture's (USDA) Food Pyramid. The differences between these two food pyramids are the following, with the AHA food pyramid putting:

- Nuts and dry beans in the meat group

- Sweet potato in the vegetable group

- Beans and white potatoes in the bread, cereal, rice, dry beans, and pasta group

- Fat-free/non-fat/low-fat milk and dairy products in the milk products group

- Eggs are removed from the meat, poultry and fish group since egg yolks are high in cholesterol

- Sodium is limited to 2400 milligrams per day

Overall, AHA recommends going easy on saturated fats, trans fats, oils, salt, and excess sugar. By reducing or eliminating saturated fat, carbohydrates make up a more significant percentage of daily intake, up to 55–60 percent, or more, of total calories.

This eating plan focuses on complex carbohydrates, such as vegetables, fruits, and grains, that contribute valuable fiber to the diet. You should regulate or minimize the amount of simple carbohydrates you get, such as sugars. That includes corn syrup, the increased consumption of which is increasingly being correlated with the rapid increase in diabetes, at least in the US. In order to get necessary nutrients, eat a variety of foods from each section of the food pyramid.

Worth noting is that the USDA Food Pyramid is being updated, and the Dietary Guidelines Advisory Committee just released proposed revisions for the guidelines. The proposed guidelines are now available for public comment for a few months prior to adoption and revision of the pyramid. These new guidelines are sensible and very heart-healthy, and are much closer to the AHA recommendations than the previous guidelines were. You can find the current (2000) guidelines at http://www.health.gov/dietaryguidelines/ and the proposed (2005) guidelines at http://www.health.gov/dietaryguidelines/dga2005/report/. The web site for the proposed guidelines has all the food and nutrition details you could want, including some excellent tables listing food sources for vitamins, minerals, and other dietary components.

The big news is that the committee recommended a decrease in grain consumption, and an increase in fruits, vegetables, dairy, and fish. The major focus of the new guidelines is to moderate your food intake based on daily caloric needs, and the higher fruit, vegetable, and dairy recommendations are to help meet our needs for specific vitamins and minerals.

For women, who typically consume 1,400 to 1,800 calories per day, this puts the recommendation for grains at 5–6 servings per day (1-ounce servings), fruits at 3 servings per day, vegetables at 3–5 servings per day, low-fat or fat-free dairy at 2–3 servings per day, lean meat and beans at 4–5 ounces per day, and oils, which should be seriously limited, at no more than 18–22 grams per day. Mayo Clinic's Food and Nutrition Center provides a useful photo guide to serving sizes for different food types, which is available at http://www.mayoclinic.com/findinformation/conditioncenters/centers.cfm?objectid=000851 DA-6222-1B37-8D7E80C8D77A0000.

Included in the meat recommendation is to consume two servings per week of fish, which contains healthy Omega-3 fatty acids. Due to the concern over heavy metals in fish, the committee recommends that pregnant women and children avoid fish with high mercury content, and that others exercise caution.

One of the most interesting departures from previous guidelines was splitting vegetables into five categories and providing weekly recommendations as some groups are too small to consume daily. For women, a 1,400 to 1,800 calorie diet would contain 1½–3 cups per week of dark-green vegetables, 1–2 cups per week of orange vegetables, 1–3 cups of legumes, 2½–3 cups of starchy vegetables, and 4½–6½ cups of other vegetables, with the lower number being for a 1,400 calorie diet and the higher number for an 1,800 calorie diet.

Using the AHA recommendations and the proposed new USDA guidelines, here are some recommendations for healthy eating, based on a 1,400 to 1,800 calorie diet. These recommendations are summarized in Figure 16.4.

Breads, cereals, and pasta: This group provides an important source of beneficial fiber, and includes both whole grains and other grains. You should get 5–6 servings, of 1-ounce each, leaning more towards whole grains due to their higher fiber content. Whole grains products include whole wheat and rye breads, whole grain/oat cereals and crackers, and brown rice. While you can consume white rice and white flour breads, crackers, cereals, and pasta, for optimal nutrition you should limit them to one-half or one-third of your daily intake. One serving could be a slice of bread, ½ cup cooked rice or pasta, ½ cup hot cereal, or 1 cup flaked cereal.

Fruits: Fruits are a very important source of vitamins, minerals, and fiber. Fresh and dried fruits are quite low in calories and have no cholesterol. It's best to minimize juices and canned fruits with added sugar. Get 3 servings per day (½ cup each). A serving is 1 small piece of fruit or ½ cup fruit juice.

Vegetables: Vegetables are also a very important source of vitamins, minerals, and fiber, and tend to be low in calories and have no cholesterol. Get 3–5 servings per day (½ cup each) selected from the five categories of vegetables. Overall, you should have the following amounts of each vegetable category each week: dark green, 1½–3 cups; orange, 1–2 cups; legumes, 1–3 cups; starchy, 2½–3 cups; and other, 4½–6½ cups. A serving is ½ cup cooked or raw vegetables or 1 cup of leafy salad greens. (See Figure 16.4 for examples of each vegetable category.)

Meat, poultry, fish, nuts, and seeds: This group is a great source of protein, but those items from animals contain cholesterol and saturated fats so stick with lean or low-fat choices. Get 4–5 ounces per day. Note that while some nuts, such as walnuts, almonds, and pecans, are high in healthy Omega-3 fatty acids, other nuts, such as cashews and macadamias, are so high in fats that they should perhaps fall into the fats and oils category.

Milk, yogurt, and cheese: While the proposed USDA guidelines recommend 2–3 cups per day of fat-free dairy for a 1,400–1,800 calorie diet, the AHA recommendations vary by age: for ages 19–50, 3 servings per day; for ages 51 and over, 4 servings per day; and for women who are pregnant or nursing, 3–4 servings per day. A serving can be 1 cup of fat-free or low-fat milk, 1 ounce low-fat cheese, ½ cup low-fat cottage cheese, or 1 cup low-fat or no-fat yogurt. For anything other than fat-free, the proposed USDA guidelines say that the difference comes out of your daily discretionary calories (see USDA proposed 2005 guidelines, referenced above, for details). Going with fat-free dairy products not only lowers your fat intake, but also your cholesterol intake.

Eggs: While they are rich in protein, B vitamins, and minerals, eggs are also high in cholesterol. AHA recommends limiting cholesterol to 300 milligrams per day, and one large egg is 213 mg. For those at risk, one egg may be too much. The cholesterol is in the yolk, with none in the egg whites, so egg whites are perfectly acceptable.

Fats and Oils: These are limited as this group is dense in calories, and solid fats are especially bad for your heart. The proposed USDA guidelines separate these into oils and solid fats. *Oils* are monounsaturated fats and polyunsaturated fats (we'll discuss these fats in more detail in the next section), and are necessary as they have essential fatty acids. Your body needs 18–22 grams of oils per day. For comparison purposes, olive oil is 14 grams per tablespoon. *Solid fats*, in contrast, are typically saturated fat or trans fat, and are considered discretionary calories, having no real nutritional value. The solid fat allowance is to accommodate anything that is not in the lowest fat form, such as milk fat in regular or low-fat dairy products, solid margarine or shortening, or meat and poultry fats. Presuming that you split your discretionary calories between solid fat and sugar, you are allowed about 12–14 grams per day of solid fats, and more if you forgo your sugar allowance of 5–8 teaspoons. While 30–36 grams per day total fat sounds like a lot of fat and oil to me as I'm on a very low-fat diet, the typical fast food meal frequently exceeds twice your daily fat and oil allowance.

Figure 16.4, below, summarizes these recommendations.

If starting on this plan is just too onerous, or if you absolutely can't do it, then simply add some fruits, vegetables, and grains to your eating each day, and that can start cutting your risk right away.

Healthy Eating Recommendations	
Food Groups	Recommended Daily Intake For 1,400–1,800 Calorie Diet
Breads, cereals, and pasta	5–6 (1-oz) servings
Fruits	3 (½ cup) servings
Vegetables, made up of: Dark-green: 1½–3 cups/week (broccoli, spinach, collards, turnips, romaine) Orange: 1–2 cups/week (carrots, sweet potatoes, squash, pumpkin) Legumes: 1–3 cups/week (pinto beans, kidney beans, peas, lentils, tofu) Starchy: 2½–3 cups/week (potatoes, corn, green peas) Other: 4½–6½ cups/week (tomatoes, lettuce, green beans, onions)	3–5 (½ cup) servings (from 5 vegetable categories)
Meat, poultry, fish, nuts, and seeds	4–5 oz
Milk, yogurt, and cheese	2–3 cups (fat-free)
Eggs	0–1 egg (if at risk, whites only)
Fats and oils Oils: 18–22 grams Solid fats: 12–14 grams	30–36 grams (see oil and solid fat details)
Discretionary calories (for sugar, and solid fat above)	See USDA 2005 Guidelines for details and allowances

Figure 16.4: Healthy Eating Recommendations

One of the biggest challenges of healthy eating is understanding fats and oils and knowing which are OK and which you should minimize or avoid, so let's delve deeper into the good, the bad, and the ugly when it comes to fats.

Fats: The Good, The Bad, and The Ugly

Are there good fats? Which fats are bad? Let's answer those questions by looking at the three major categories of fats: saturated fats, trans fats (hybrid), and unsaturated fats. Of the unsaturated fats, there are two kinds: polyunsaturated fats and monounsaturated fats.

1) **Good: Unsaturated fats** (oils) are liquid at room temperature

- **Polyunsaturated fats** are also liquid in the refrigerator. They include safflower, sesame, sunflower, corn, soybean, and some nut oils. Polyunsaturated fats help the body remove cholesterol, reducing buildup in the arteries.

- **Monounsaturated fats** start becoming solid when refrigerated. They include canola, olive, and peanut oils, as well as avocados. Monounsaturated fats can also help reduce cholesterol if used in conjunction with a diet low in saturated fats.

2) **Bad: Saturated fats** are high in cholesterol, and are usually solid, even at room temperature. They generally come from animal sources, such as beef, lamb, pork, butter, cream, milk, cheese, and yogurt, but may also come from some plant sources, such as coconut oil, palm oil, and palm kernel oil. Food labels on processed foods indicate the amount of saturated fat they contain.

3) **Ugly: Trans fats** are the secret, hidden fats commonly found in baked goods and processed foods. They are not currently shown on food labels, but must be by 2006. Fortunately, many food companies are way ahead in reformulating their products to remove the trans fats so they don't have to show them on labels. Why are trans fats so ugly? They are created by taking good fats (liquid) and turning them into bad ones (solid) through hydrogenation, the adding of hydrogen atoms to oils. This makes them shelf-stable to stay fresh longer and solidifies the fat to improve the texture of processed foods (think Oreo crème). Trans fats raise total cholesterol levels, raise bad LDL cholesterol, and lower good HDL cholesterol, all of which increase the risk of heart disease. Foods high in trans fats include French fries, donuts, cookies, and crackers, which you should avoid when possible. There are now cookies and crackers on the market that contain absolutely no trans fats, so look for them, but read the labels with care. Be prepared to accept a change in texture to eliminate the trans fats. Even Oreos are being reformulated, with the new golden Oreos being free of trans fats.

Recommendation

Unsaturated fats are preferable to saturated fats and trans fats, with the AHA recommending 40 per cent polyunsaturated fats and 60 per cent monounsaturated fats.

What about the controversy between butter and margarine? Stick margarines have trans fats, and butter is rich in artery-clogging saturated fat and cholesterol. Which is the better choice? Neither, actually. Margarines made from vegetable oils, such as canola, contain no dietary cholesterol, and the more liquid they are, the less trans fats. The best bet then is diet or light margarine, which has less trans fat, and in some cases is trans fat-free. Look for one that has no more than 2 grams of saturated fat per tablespoon and for which vegetable oil is the first ingredient.

There are also new plant-derived spreads (Take Control and Benecol) that have been shown to lower cholesterol by up to 10 per cent by keeping the body from absorbing the cholesterol from other foods. In addition, there are fat-free, heart-healthy squeezable margarine products, though they are not for use in cooking. A small amount of olive oil is also fine. Of course, you can always just give up butter and margarine, which I've mostly done and don't miss them.

Let's explore some other details related to food groups.

Fruits and Vegetables

A study done by the National Heart, Lung, and Blood Institute found that the higher the consumption of fruits and vegetables, the lower the LDL cholesterol level. That applied to both women and men. Based on their results, eating five or more servings per day of fruits and vegetables could decrease your risk of heart disease by 12–15 per cent. Corroborating that, the study at McMaster University mentioned earlier pointed out that getting adequate fruits and vegetables can yield as much as a thirty per cent decrease in heart attack risk.

Fiber

Another vital category in a heart-healthy diet is fiber. I figure that's one of the secrets to my weight loss success.

There are some interesting data points related to fiber from the American Association of Nutritional Sciences (http://www.nutrition.org/). A study presented at their conference showed that analyzing data from a US Department of Agriculture study into the consumption of whole grains yielded the following correlation: women consuming three or more servings per day of whole grain products had a significantly lower body mass index (BMI) than those who ate less than one serving per day. While we don't know whether eating whole grains helps keep the fat off, or if those who focus on getting whole grains are also focused on controlling their weight and health, it is still an interesting data point.

Other studies have shown that increased consumption of dietary fiber indeed appears to decrease the risk of getting cardiovascular diseases and Type 2 diabetes. A diet rich in whole grains appears to be useful in controlling weight and reducing your risk of illness.

One of my favorite fiber sources is flaxseed because it is a good source of helpful Omega-3 fatty acids. For more details on flaxseed, see the story in Figure 16.5.

Flaxseed: Could It End Bad Hair Days?

I was consulting with my friend, Natalie Elliott, about nutrition. She is a clinical nutritionist and the owner of Brainwaves Music and Wellness here in Austin. "Do you have a fatty-acid imbalance?" she asked.

"What is a fatty-acid imbalance? Is it related to those Omega-3 fatty acids which we hear so much about?" I asked. "Yes," she replied.

"How do you know if you have an imbalance?" I asked. She said that skin and hair can be indicators—if you have dry or scaly skin, soft or brittle nails, or unmanageable hair, you just might have a fatty-acid imbalance. Who would have thought that a fatty-acid imbalance could cause bad-hair days?

Other indicators include excessive thirst, frequent infections, poor wound healing, dry eyes, irritability, hyperactivity, weakness, or fatigue. I'll admit to having the dry skin, soft nails, and much too-frequent bad-hair days.

She continued to talk about Omega-3 fatty acids and Omega-6 fatty acids, saying, "Our bodies need at least a 1:3 ratio (1:1 is better) of Omega-3 to Omega-6, but most Americans have about a 1:20 ratio because of the fats we use in cooking. As a result, we tend to have severe fatty-acid imbalances." Why is that a problem? A fatty-acid

Flaxseed: Could It End Bad Hair Days?

imbalance has been correlated with cancer, heart disease, and other issues.

Omega-6 fatty acids are the bad guys and are called "sticky, clumpy fats." While they lower the bad cholesterol (LDL), they also lower the good cholesterol, thus increasing your risk of heart disease. The American Heart Association reports a link between high Omega-6 intake and sudden death from heart attacks. Omega-6 fatty acids include common oils used in cooking, such as corn oil, cottonseed oil, safflower oil, soybean oil, and squeeze margarines.

In contrast, Omega-3s are the good guys and are important in our diets according to nutritionists, who point out that this information isn't well known, even among doctors. They say that Omega-3 fatty acids lower the bad (LDL) cholesterol, raise the good (HDL) cholesterol, and reduce the inflammation of the arteries that otherwise leads to heart disease. In addition, Omega-3s keep the blood platelets from being so sticky, thus reducing the risk of blood clots and build-up in the blood vessels. Cultures with high Omega-3 intake have low incidence of heart disease and diabetes. And Omega-3 also helps decrease arthritis.

Omega-3s are found in fatty fish, such as salmon, tuna, and mackerel. The American Heart Association says we should eat two servings of these each week, and some nutritionists say we should have a serving every day. But, there is concern over the safety of fish due to the occasional presence of heavy metals in their flesh.

For those of you, like me, who are allergic to fish, there is still hope. Omega-3 is also available in nuts, olives, olive oil, dark leafy-green vegetables, avocados, and flaxseed.

You've never heard of flaxseed? Nutritionists are very big on it. Natalie, my nutritionist friend, says that flaxseed is an ancient grain that was so highly regarded in Egypt that it was buried with the pharaohs to assure them of a healthy afterlife. Flaxseed has a higher level of Omega-3 than fish, also contains lignins, which appear to reduce the incidence of breast and prostate cancer, and is high in soluble and insoluble fiber, which helps prevent colon cancer.

Most of us need only 2 tablespoons per day of ground flaxseed, which you can add to your breakfast cereal for a nutty taste, or sprinkle over other foods. Those with heart and other diseases can benefit from 4–6 tablespoons per day.

A friend was recently commenting that his wife was reluctant to eat flaxseed as she was concerned that it would change the taste of her foods. But after trying it, she was surprised at how much she liked the mild, slightly nutty flavor of flaxseed. I agree. I've developed a taste for it, and I know it's good for my health.

Flaxseed could well cure your fatty-acid imbalance. Just think about it: in addition to keeping you healthy, it might even put an end to "bad-hair days".

Figure 16.5: Flaxseed: Could It End Bad Hair Days?

Beverages

Though the AHA and USDA food pyramids don't speak specifically to beverages other than milk, and alcohol as part of the discretionary calorie allowance, beverages are still an important part of a heart-healthy diet. Here are a few data points related to beverages.

Fat-free milk: From my own experience, I'd recommend not making the change from regular milk to low-fat or fat-free milk by going cold-turkey. I had to, since disgusting fat-free skim milk was all that the hospital served me. When I got home and had organic fat-free milk, it tasted wonderful by comparison. You, however, may want to make the transition gradually so that you can adjust at each step of the way, and the change will therefore be less noticeable.

Hydration: The Institute of Medicine (http://www.iom.edu/), created by the US government, proclaimed that the need for eight glasses of water each day is a myth and says that you get enough fluid by drinking when thirsty. Contrary to what we've always been told, they say, coffee, milk, fruits, vegetables, and other beverages really do contribute to our fluid needs. Water is vital to your health, but you can get it from lots of sources. Just be careful of the sugar content of juices and other beverages.

Coffee: While coffee has been exonerated of causing heart disease and pancreatic cancer, the jury is still out on whether it is linked to hypertension, though most studies haven't found a link. The hypothesis that coffee may increase blood cholesterol also hasn't been proven. Recently, a Finnish study that was reported in the New England Journal of Medicine indicated that coffee even reduces the risk of Type 2 diabetes.

Alcohol: Does alcohol play a role in heart disease? My doctor recommended a glass of wine (or similar drink) each day to keep the blood vessels open and to minimize stress. Several studies have also found a reduction of heart attack risk from drinking alcohol. The study at McMaster University pointed out that consuming alcohol in moderation decreased the risk of heart attacks by nine per cent. And in what could be heralded as good news for beer drinkers, Japanese researchers reported in the International Journal of Cancer that rats receiving beer showed a reduced risk of colon cancer. (This scenario conjures up some interesting images.) Beer is high in antioxidants, and may be found to have similar effects to red wine. Neither alcohol, nor hops, provided the same protective effect. I'm not recommending that you start drinking, but be aware of the findings and discuss this with your doctor.

My Diet Experiences

As I mentioned, I am on a fat-free diet to avoid the further buildup of plaque in my arteries and to lose weight. Even before my surgery, I ate a healthy diet—organics at home, and on the road when I could find them, lots of fresh fruits and vegetables, and no fried foods. However, my weakness was dairy products, so I've now removed all dairy fats by switching to fat-free milk, cheese, sour cream, and yogurt.

For me, the biggest adjustment wasn't moving to fat-free dairy, but instead was adding bread and grains to my diet. I've never really cared for bread—I can take it or leave it—so for me that was hard.

Surprisingly, I don't miss the fats in my diet. Foods seem to taste fresher and healthier. With no fats, there's no more heartburn. I've lost weight and feel much better. Eating heart-smart also helps avoid other health issues, such as colon cancer.

That didn't mean I couldn't have any fat—it just meant that my diet had to be extremely low in fat. I had to avoid the bad fats (saturated and trans fats), but can eat small quantities of good ones.

On this journey, I've found some wonderful foods that have helped me immensely by making a fat-free diet easier, and in some cases even enjoyable. After all, every woman needs chocolate sometimes, and who would have thought you could find fat-free brownies and cookies. I've included in Figure 16.6 some of my secrets, favorite resources, and tips for staying on a low-fat diet. If you find others that help you, please write and let me know about them.

My Low-Fat/Fat-Free Eating Secrets

Fruits and vegetables (fresh or frozen, or canned with no added sugar) are fat-free and should be the largest component in the diet. They are a given, so I'm not going to discuss them here. What I've included in this table are things that I've discovered can help you stick to a low-fat or fat-free diet. Since most of us are time-starved, I've included prepared and convenience foods here that can supplement your diet.

Sweets

First, the important stuff, sweets. That's the hardest part about dieting. Don't you just occasionally want a cookie or brownie? I had mostly given up dessert, especially chocolate, but medical science has recently discovered that chocolate, in moderation, is good for your heart. That's especially true of dark chocolate, which is full of flavonoids. Here are my diet dessert solutions:

❑ No Pudge Fudge Brownies–awesome brownies that even my teenage son loves. You make them with fat-free yogurt instead of oil. If you don't find them at your local store, ask for them, or order online. Flavors: Original, Raspberry, Cappuccino, and Mint (wonderful). (See Appendix B for Resources.)

❑ Joseph's Fat-Free Cookies–only 20 calories apiece (they're small). Order online, with free shipping. Flavors: Chocolate Chocolate Chip, Ginger, and Mint Chocolate (my favorite). (See Appendix B for Resources.)

❑ Newman's Own Fat-Free Fig Newtons—no fat, very satisfying, and 60 calories apiece. Whole Foods 365 Brand Organic Fig Bars are similar. (Note: Whole Foods brands are only available at Whole Foods Markets, headquartered in Austin—see http://www.wholefoods.com/ for locations in 29 US states, Canada, and the UK.)

❑ Meringue cookies – available at stores, or make your own.

❑ Make your own treat – mix walnuts (full of good Omega-3 fatty acids) and raisins or another dried fruit (very good for you), eat, and enjoy. This feels sinful, even if it isn't. Dark fruits, such as raisins, blueberries, cranberries, dates, and figs, are especially protective for your heart. This is a good, heart-healthy emergency food for travel.

My Low-Fat/Fat-Free Eating Secrets
Dairy

Here are some of the fat-free and low-fat dairy products that we use. We have tried some products that we didn't like, and there are many others that we haven't yet tried because they aren't in our stores or we just liked the product that we tried first.

Fat free milk works well for cooking, but many of the other fat-free products do not. Cheeses will soften on top of hot foods, but don't cook well. We use the milk, half and half, and yogurts below, in conjunction with fruits, to whip up fat-free frozen yogurts and ice creams.

❑   Organic Valley or Horizon Fat-Free Milk—zero fat.

❑   Land O'Lakes Fat-Free Half and Half—zero fat and 20 calories per tablespoon. It adds richness to coffee or low-fat cream sauces.

❑   Kraft Fat-Free Cheddar and Mozzarella—zero fat and 45 calories per ¼ cup. We use the mozzarella for making healthy home-made pizza.

❑   Kraft Fat-Free Slices in Cheddar and Swiss—zero fat and 30 calories per slice.

❑   Lifetime Cheddar, Swiss, and Monterey Jack—zero fat and 40 calories per 1" cube.

❑   Organic Valley Low-fat Sour Cream—1.25 grams of fat per tablespoon.

❑   Philadelphia Fat-Free Cream Cheese—zero fat and 20 calories per tablespoon. Works great for making fat-free creamed spinach—even my teenage son loves it.

❑   Cascade Fresh and Horizon Fat-Free Yogurts—zero fat, with plain being 160–170 calories per cup and flavors being 110–130 calories for ¾ cup. Plain is great for cooking and the flavors are great for making frozen yogurt.

❑   Smart Squeeze Non-Fat Margarine Spread—squeezable butter substitute with zero fat and 5 calories per tablespoon. Don't use for cooking—use oil instead.

❑   Egg white products—zero fat. There are many brands (Egg Beaters, etc.) for making omelets and using in place of eggs.

Grains

❑   Kashi Heart-to-Heart Oat Cereal—1.5 grams of fat and 110 calories per ¾ cup. It's called a Healthy Heart System because in addition to oats and other whole grains, it contains lots of heart-healthy nutrition, including antioxidants, vitamins E and C, beta carotene, lycopene, B vitamins, soluble fiber, green tea, and grape seed extract. There is also a great looking brownie recipe using this cereal on the Kashi web site, at http://www.kashi.com, at the bottom of the page.

❑   Kashi Strawberry Fields cereal—zero fat and 120 calories per cup. It's a rice cereal with dried strawberries and raspberries.

❑   There are lots of other low-fat cereals that you can try, but many of them contain soy, to which I'm allergic, so I haven't tried them and can't make recommendations.

My Low-Fat/Fat-Free Eating Secrets

❑ Ground flaxseed is a major source of heart-healthy Omega-3 fatty acids, with 3 grams of fat per tablespoon. This is particularly good for those who cannot eat fish. I add flaxseed to my breakfast cereal to get extra fiber and Omega-3 fatty acids, and also sprinkle it over other dishes for added fiber. There are several brands of ground flaxseed, and some are fortified with additional vitamins. You can also get flaxseed meal, such as Bob's Red Mill brand, for adding to things that you cook. (See Figure 16.5 for more about flaxseed)

❑ Whole Foods Flaxseed Bread—one gram of fat and 120 calories per slice. It contains no saturated fat and no added oil, with all fat being from the flaxseed. An excellent source of fiber, it contains whole wheat and rye in addition to flaxseed.

❑ Lots of breads, especially French and sour dough, have no oil, so are good for fat-free diets.

❑ Up Country Naturals Vermont Baking Mix—zero fat and 70 calories per serving. When in a hurry, we have used this for biscuits by not adding oil, and it was quite good. It can also be used for waffles, muffins, and pancakes, perhaps without adding egg, oil, or butter, or by adding only minute quantities or using Egg Beaters. Obviously, you can make these from scratch as well.

❑ Whole Foods Fat-Free Flour Tortillas—zero fat and 145 calories each.

❑ Whole Foods 365 Brand Baked Woven Wheat Crackers—zero fat (0.5 grams for 8 crackers, all monounsaturated) and 15 calories per cracker.

❑ Kashi TLC crackers—about 1 gram fat for about 5–6 crackers (3 grams fat for 15–18 crackers, depending on flavor) and 7–9 calories per cracker. These crackers have no trans fats. Flavors: Original 7-Grain, Honey Sesame, Cheddar, and Natural Ranch.

❑ Most wheat pasta and rice noodles (Pad Thai, etc.) are fat free or low fat, and some are made with whole grains that provide lots of fiber. Topping a small serving of pasta with diced tomatoes, onions, mushrooms, and olives makes for a heart-healthy Mediterranean-style dish.

Snacks

  ❑ Nuts, such as walnuts, almonds, and pecans, are healthy fats and make a good snack. Be aware that cashews and macadamias are high in fat.

  ❑ Nature's Choice Cereal Bars in Multigrain Triple Berry and Apple Cinnamon—1.5 grams of fat and 120 calories each. You can stash these in your purse or computer bag for emergency meals, but be aware that they are crumbly. If you're not allergic to soy (as I am), then protein bars also make good emergency meals.

  ❑ Frito Lay baked chips—Baked Original Potato Crisps are 1.5 grams of fat and 110 calories for about 11 chips, and Baked Tostitos are 1 gram of fat and 110 calories for about 20 chips.

My Low-Fat/Fat-Free Eating Secrets

❑ Newman's Own Pretzel Sticks (and other pretzels) are 1 gram of fat and 110 calories for about 13 pretzel sticks. Most brands of pretzels are very low fat.

Soups

❑ Fat-free broths, such as Health Valley and Whole Foods Market 365 Brand (in aseptic packages that keep well in the pantry), come in chicken, vegetable, and beef, and make a good soup starter. Add leftover meat chunks, veggies, rice, or pasta for a quick fat-free or low-fat-soup.

Dressings and Condiments

❑ The Silver Palate's Low-Fat Roasted Garlic Balsamic Salad Splash—1 gram of fat and 20 calories per tablespoon, and Lemon Garlic Herb Salad Splash—1 gram of fat and 15 calories per tablespoon both work well on green salads and for making pasta salads.

❑ Fat-free condiments include salsa, pickles, mustards, ketchups, and some barbecue sauces.

Eating Out

Eating out isn't always easy on a fat-free diet, and most low-fat menu items are more than my whole day's allowance of fats. However, restaurants are generally quite flexible and willing to accommodate, so I simply order what it is that I can eat.

❑ Most restaurants can prepare grilled chicken and steamed veggies, made with no fats, so that's a consistent choice. (Fish is also a good choice.)

❑ A salad with lots of veggies is another good choice, especially with grilled chicken or shrimp. Some restaurants have good fat-free dressings—Chili's has fat-free honey mustard and Outback has fat-free French. You can also try olive oil and vinegar, or worst case, lemon juice.

❑ Subway has "7 under 6" salads and subs, ranging from 2 to 6 grams of fat.

❑ If a restaurant can't accommodate me (it hasn't happened yet), then I always have my emergency food stash to fall back on.

Figure 16.6: My Low-Fat/Fat-Free Eating Secrets

Today, having been on a very-low-fat diet, I don't want stuff that's high in fat. My stomach knots up at the thought of cheesecake and other fattening foods. In fact, I've found that you can make truly delightful low-fat cuisine.

Diet Challenges

Of course, being on a special diet has its own set of challenges, especially in restaurants and on the road. A fat-free diet means never ordering straight from a restaurant menu again. But I've yet to find a restaurant that wasn't willing to accommodate my special needs.

It's a bit harder in airports, but if I can't find salads with grilled chicken, I always have my emergency stash of food—cereal bars, crackers, dried fruits and nuts.

Until recently, I had felt that most fast food wasn't heart healthy, but I've learned differently through my work with the American Heart Association's Heart Walk. Subway, a national presenting sponsor of the Heart Walk, has focused on creating lots of heart-healthy food choices, and through a friend there, I've had my eyes opened to a whole new array of low-fat foods. Subway's "7 under 6" foods include sandwiches and salads with lean meats and having only minimal fats, generally 6 grams or less, and in many cases as low as 2–4 grams. Best of all, they carry two kinds of fat-free dressings, whereas most fast food restaurants don't even carry one low-fat dressing, much less fat-free.

Subway has a nutritionist on staff and posts nutrition details on the web site (http://www.subway.com/applications/NutritionInfo/index.aspx). Look for foods labeled "6 grams of fat or less". With Subway focused so heavily on healthy kids through the Subway FRESH Steps childhood obesity initiative, it's a place where you can teach kids about living a healthy life. I was impressed with the healthy eating information on Subway's web site, including providing information for people with food allergies.

When I attend conferences and banquets, my special diet is a challenge—it means always getting my grilled chicken and steamed broccoli when everyone else is having dessert or coffee, and never getting dessert. At the banquet at a recent conference, when the waiter presented me raspberry sorbet for dessert, I was thrilled and thanked him profusely for my first "non-chicken dessert"!

Sometimes language plays havoc with special meals. At one conference, the waiter went to get my fat-free meal, showing up as dessert was served with a glass of fat-free milk! Note to self: Learn "fat-free meal" in Spanish. For my recent trip to Italy, the first Italian I learned was "senza grassi"—no fat.

Speaking of that trip, we had fun juggling multiple diets. It was four girls (Mother, my sisters, Stephanie and Tracy, and me) and four different diets—fat-free, Atkins, The Zone, and for our skinny little mother, the "whatever no one else wants" diet. To make the special diets easier to deal with since we weren't fluent in Italian, I traded in hotel points for upgrades to the executive floor—with breakfast each morning in the concierge lounge, and appetizers, pizza, and beverages there in the evenings, we ate just a single meal out each day. In restaurants, we either requested special preparation using our limited Italian, or simply swapped around foods based on what each could eat. That worked fine.

Now that I'm eating right, and eating regularly, which was hard to do when I was constantly on the road and in meetings, my stress level has come way down.

Lest you think I'm blowing smoke talking about diet, let me assure you that I know just how difficult it is to lose weight. Before my heart problems, I had lost 22 pounds over several months, so it wasn't a fast weight loss. Since coming out of the hospital last year, I've lost

63 more pounds, for a total of 85 pounds. It's not easy for me to admit that I needed to lose that much, but it's a fact, so I might as well accept it and admit it.

Over the years, I've done lots of diets, complete with the yo-yo effect. Diets never seemed to make a permanent change. This time, though, the change is permanent because I've changed my eating habits and I have the incentive. Now, I truly do eat to live, and know that tripping up could be fatal.

The bottom line is that if I can do it, I know you can, too, because I'm sure that you have much more willpower than I did. There is something, besides the fat-free diet, that made it a whole lot easier. My weight loss started as a result of listening to a program called *Achieve Your Chosen Weight* (tape/CD). I'm usually skeptical about that kind of thing, but something told me to do this, and it worked.

It reprogrammed my eating, causing me to drop the weight. It was easy. It helped me get over having to clean my plate. When you were little, were you told to clean your plate because there were starving children in Asia or Europe? Many of us were. It's time to forget that. Plates today are huge, especially when we go out to eat. They are much too full, and we shouldn't eat it all. It's enough to feed you for two meals or more, so that's exactly what I do with it—I eat some, and take the rest home for another meal or two.

The key to losing weight is to shrink your stomach, and this program helped me to do that by resetting my eating. I listen to it as I go to sleep at night and to continue to reinforce my new habits. Between this and the fat-free diet, it has been surprisingly easy to lose 85 pounds. In case you're interested, you'll find more information in Appendix B. By the way, in that same series you'll find other helpful titles, such as *Relieve Stress*, *Restful Sleep*, *Relax and Succeed*, *Overcome Anxiety*, and more. If I can do it, I know you can, too.

The Downside of Losing Weight

Of course, losing weight does have a downside—clothes. I've had lots of closet issues from losing so many sizes, meaning that I've had to replace my wardrobe several times in the span of about 18 months. I had a few things still stashed away in my closet from when I went up in weight and was able to wear them for a while as I came down, but it's all too big now.

Fortunately, my sister, Tracy, owns four designer consignment boutiques (the good news); unfortunately, she lives about 1,000 miles away, in Birmingham, so I only get there a few times a year.

As you're losing weight, you can look for a consignment shop in your area to sell those clothes that you can no longer wear and to bridge the gap as you're going down. Tracy belongs to, and has just assumed the presidency of, the National Association of Resale and Thrift Shops (http://www.narts.org/shopping/), which provides a search of member stores, as shown in Figure 16.7. You can search by state, area code, or category (ladies, junior, formal, etc.) to find consignment shops in your area. It's a good resource.

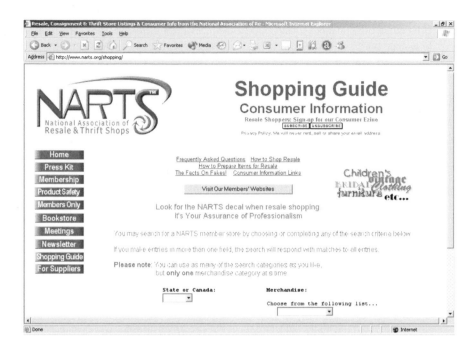

Figure 16.7: Consignment Shop Search at the National Association of Resale and Thrift Shops (http://www.narts.org/shopping/)

If you're near Birmingham, look Tracy up at Collage Designer Consignment Boutique. Her web site (http://www.shopcollage.com) is shown in Figure 16.8. Collage was voted the #1 Women's Boutique and the #1 Consignment Shop in Birmingham Magazine, and was chosen the 2003 Retailer of the Year by the Alabama Retail Association.

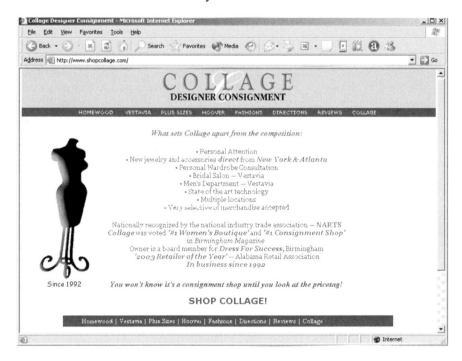

Figure 16.8: Collage Designer Consignment Boutique, if you're near Birmingham, Alabama (http://www.shopcollage.com)

And while I'm bragging, let me also brag about my other sister, Stephanie, a graphic artist and branding expert. Stephanie did Tracy's web site and she designed my web site, marketing materials, and the gorgeous cover for this book.

Creating Your Plan For Healthy Eating

In this chapter, you learned about various types of diets, got suggestions for heart-healthy eating, and read about what diets worked for other women. Now it's time to take all the input about diet and healthy eating and decide what it means for you, creating your plan for healthy eating.

We'll take the steps related to healthy eating that you decided to accomplish in Figure 15.2 and break them into more detail so that you can implement them. Let's start by answering the questions below.

1) What is my eating normally like? Am I on a diet? If so, which one? How is it working for me?

2) What is my goal, what do I hope to accomplish, or how will I benefit? Some examples might be:

- Lose weight: If so, how much?

- Control cholesterol: If so, what's my goal?

- Manage blood pressure: If so, what my goal?

3) What are my options for accomplishing my goals, and what are the pros and cons of each?

4) What kind of eating plan will I commit to? What steps and interim stages will I commit to?

As an example, in Figure 16.9, I answered these questions as I would answer them now.

Goals for Healthy Eating

1. What is my eating normally like? Am I on a diet? If so, which one? How is it working for me?

   I'm now on a fat-free/low-fat diet, by doctor's orders. I have lost weight on this diet, though my weight is currently plateaued. I avoid fried foods, fast foods, and high-fat foods. I eat lots of raw and cooked fruits and vegetables. I used to avoid bread and grains as a waste of perfectly good calories but have added them back as a necessary source of fiber. I limit my dairy to fat-free products. I limit my quantities of food, and don't worry about finishing everything on my plate.

2. What is my goal, what do I hope to accomplish, or how will I benefit?

I need to continue to lose X pounds to get down to XXX pounds. I need to maintain my low blood pressure and cholesterol, and to increase my good HDL cholesterol.

3. What are my options for accomplishing my goals, and what are the pros and cons of each?

    There are no other options – it's fat-free for me, by doctor's orders.

4. What kind of eating plan will I commit to? What steps and interim stages will I commit to?

    I will maintain a fat-free/low-fat version of the Healthy Eating Plan (like the one in Figure 16.4). I will minimize the quantity of saturated fats through rigorously managing portions, using only fat-free dairy products, and keeping the quantity of red meats I eat closely controlled. I need to balance the amount of seafood, poultry, and lean meats in my diet. I need to ensure that I get sufficient servings of cereals and grains as well as fresh fruits and vegetables. Though I get lots of water, I could probably get more to stay even better hydrated. And under doctor's orders, I get a glass of alcohol each day. And on some occasions, I let myself have tiny amounts of chocolate.

Figure 16.9: Sample Goals for Healthy Eating

Take a moment now to answer these same questions for you, in Figure 16.10, based on your current situation and using as input your plan from Figure 15.2.

Goals for Healthy Eating

1. What is my eating normally like? Am I on a diet? If so, which one? How is it working for me?

2. What is my goal, what do I hope to accomplish, or how will I benefit?

3. What are my options for accomplishing my goals, and what are the pros and cons of each?

4. What kind of eating plan will I commit to? What steps and interim stages will I commit to?

Figure 16.10: Your Goals for Healthy Eating

If you've decided to implement your goals using the Healthy Eating Recommendations outlined previously in Figure 16.4, then create your Healthy Eating Plan in Figure 16.11 by filling in the details about your current eating, your committed steps, and your target dates for reaching those commitments.

Healthy Eating Plan and Targets				
Food Groups	Current Servings Per Day	Ideal Servings Per Day	Commitments/ Action Steps	Target Dates
Breads, cereals, and pasta		5–6 (1-oz)		
Fruits		3 (½ c)		

Vegetables, made up of:
    Dark-green: 1½–3 c/wk
    Orange: 1–2 c/wk
    Legumes: 1–3 c/wk
    Starchy: 2½–3 c/wk
    Other: 4½–6½ c/wk
		3–5 (½ c)		

Meat, poultry, fish, nuts, and seeds		4–5 oz		
Milk, yogurt, and cheese (fat-free)		2–3 cups		
Eggs		0–1 egg		

Fats and oils
    Oils: 18–22 g
    Solid fats: 12–14 g
		30–36 g		

Discretionary calories		USDA 2005 Guidelines		

Figure 16.11: Your Healthy Eating Plan and Targets

As you're considering your new eating plan, consider whether this would be good for the whole family, especially in teaching your kids and establishing healthy eating habits for a lifetime.

As you develop your eating plan, there are lots of recent diet and healthy eating facts that may useful to you, though not to everyone. Please peruse Figure 16.12, Miscellaneous Diet and Disease Facts, and Figure 16.13, Miscellaneous Food Facts. These tables are not intended to be read as text, but simply to peruse for facts that may be relevant to you. In addition, the whole area of vitamins and minerals is an important area that I'm not specifically dealing with here because it is so individualized, but I have included some interesting facts in Figure 16.14, Miscellaneous Vitamin and Mineral Facts.

There are also a lot of resources on the web that can help you in planning and carrying out your eating plan so I've included references to some helpful resources in Figure 16.15, at the end of this chapter.

Miscellaneous Diet and Disease Facts

☐ American women consume 335 more calories per day today than twenty years ago, at almost 1,900 calories per day. Most of the increase is from soft drinks and sugary snacks, increasing the risk of diabetes. Total fat intake has remained the same.

☐ Women in the US who doubled their fiber intake from 12 grams to 24 grams per day absorbed 90 fewer calories per day from fat and protein.

☐ The Mediterranean diet reduces the risk of heart disease by reducing "inflammation-related proteins."

☐ People who had two servings per day of processed baked goods, which contain trans fats, were twice as likely to experience vision loss as those who consumed none. Those with high fat diets of 70 grams per day were at three times the risk of progressing to advanced macular degeneration. Those eating a diet high in saturated fat and trans fat increased their risk of both heart disease and macular degeneration, suggesting a link between hardening of blood vessels to the retina and hardening of arteries to heart.

☐ Those who rely more on food prepared outside the home are at risk from bigger portions, which causes more weight gain. The fewer vegetables, fruit, beans, and grains they get, the more they are at risk of cancer, heart disease, and other chronic illnesses.

☐ A study into slowing the aging process found that those on a high-nutrition, calorie-restricted diet experienced lower risk of heart disease and diabetes based on measures of cholesterol, blood pressure, fasting glucose, and insulin.

☐ Calories eaten earlier in the day are more satiating than the same calories eaten later in the day, according to research at the University of Texas at El Paso. This reinforces the old adage to eat like a king at breakfast, and like a pauper at dinner.

☐ Men get more benefit than women from a diet low in saturated fat—in women cholesterol dropped 12%, whereas in men cholesterol dropped 19%.

☐ Things that prevent colon cancer include eating whole grains, fruits, and vegetables, especially those containing phytochemicals (broccoli, cabbage, cauliflower, kale, and Brussels sprouts); avoiding saturated fats; losing weight; avoiding smoking; and keeping alcohol intake moderate.

☐ Those with four or more servings per week of beef, pork, or lamb were three times as likely to have colon cancer. However, consuming eight grams of fiber per day cut the risk in half.

☐ A study of women in Mexico that consumed high-carbohydrate diets, which were particularly high in corn products, found that they were twice as likely to get breast cancer. Researchers theorize that the carbohydrates raise blood sugar and provide an environment favorable for replication of cancer cells. Women in the study who consumed more fruits, vegetables, and whole grains, all of which contain insoluble fiber, had far less breast cancer risk, leading to speculation that diets higher in insoluble fiber put women at less risk of breast cancer. American women typically

Miscellaneous Diet and Disease Facts

consume diets that are much lower in carbohydrates than the women studied.

Figure 16.12: Miscellaneous Diet and Disease Facts

Miscellaneous Food Facts

Bread, cereal, and pasta

❑ Oats contain a soluble fiber, called beta glucan, which lowers LDL and total cholesterol and helps control blood sugar. It contains phytochemicals that reduce heart disease risk and antioxidants that relax blood vessels and maintain blood flow.

Fruits and vegetables

❑ Flavones protect against breast cancer—each 0.5 gram per day of celery, lettuce, peppers, spinach, chili pepper, lemon, or parsley decreases breast cancer risk by 13%.

❑ Fast food salads can fool you into thinking that they're low-fat or low-calorie. They can be more fattening than a burger and fries because of high-fat dressing, bacon, cheese, and croutons.

❑ Antioxidants in fruits and vegetables prevent disease by combating cell-damaging free radicals. A good source is dark fruits and vegetables, such as berries, cherries, grapes, oranges, plums, kale, peppers, red cabbage, and spinach. The highest amounts are found in pomegranate and walnuts—yet another good reason to enjoy walnuts.

❑ Tomatoes contain carotenoids, including lycopene. Cooked or processed tomatoes have more "available" lycopene, from 2–10 times as much. Women with high blood levels of lycopene had one-third less cardiovascular disease risk.

❑ Yellow corn contains the carotenoids lutein and zeaxanthin, which keep eyes healthy.

Meat, poultry, fish, nuts, and seeds

❑ Shrimp has cholesterol, so we've been steered away from it, but it is actually a healthy choice. It's low in saturated fat, which is a greater cholesterol problem than cholesterol in foods. Shrimp also contains Omega-3 fatty acids. Much shellfish is lower in cholesterol than chicken or beef.

❑ Chemicals and heavy metals in fish are a problem for pregnant women and children. Because of PCBs in farmed salmon and mercury in large fish (sword, shark, tuna, and king mackerel), various nutrition sources recommend no more than 8 ounces per month for pregnant women and children as fetal/infant brains are easily damaged by these chemicals, and for the rest of us, no more than 12 oz of fish per week and we should vary the species.

Miscellaneous Food Facts

Dairy and eggs

❏ Saturated fat and trans fat play a bigger role in raising blood cholesterol than dietary cholesterol does, so one egg is probably OK.

Fats and oils

❏ Trans fats increase fat accumulation in the waist area, increasing waist circumference.

❏ The National Heart, Lung, and Blood Institute Family Heart Study found that to reduce high triglycerides, add flaxseed, walnuts, and canola oil to the diet, all of which are rich in an Omega-3 fat that lowers triglycerides.

Beverages

❏ Moderate alcohol can be heart healthy. That's defined as 12 ounces of beer, 5 ounces of wine, or 1.5 ounces of 80-proof liquor.

❏ Tea protects against plaque in the arteries.

Miscellaneous

❏ Great news—chocolate is good for us. It is a plant, and therefore contains no cholesterol. It's full of flavonoids, an antioxidant that reduces the harmful effects of LDL. Dark chocolate has more flavonoids. Chocolate also lowers blood pressure, and decreases the growth of cancer cells. It has the same chemicals as tea, and 1 ounce of chocolate is equivalent to 1 cup of black tea. In a study, men who ate from one to three chocolate bars per month lived longer than those eating none.

Figure 16.13: Miscellaneous Food Facts

Miscellaneous Vitamin and Mineral Facts

❏ Everyone is unique in their vitamin and mineral needs. Your medical situation can create interrelationships that dictate unique needs, or even things to avoid, so this is an area to discuss with your health care provider and in which to stay updated. A couple of examples:

　○ Those on Coumadin®, a blood thinner, should steer clear of the usual recommendation to take Vitamin E due to the potential for clotting problems and excessive bleeding. Those taking full-strength aspirin or an anti-inflammatory may also be at risk.

　○ Those with stents should ignore the frequent recommendation that everyone should be taking folic acid. At the time of my heart surgery, research had shown that it was valuable for heart patients, but subsequent research has shown that folic acid has been correlated with stent failures.

❏ According to three studies (Harvard Nurses Health Study, Health Professionals Follow-Up Study, and Women's Health Study), people with the highest level of magnesium in their diets, such as from grains, fruits, vegetables, beans, and nuts, have the lowest risk of diabetes.

❑ Drinking hard water seems to reduce heart disease risk as it contains magnesium, calcium, and other minerals. Fluoride in the water also appears to reduce risk.

❑ The US Institute of Medicine reports that we need less sodium and more potassium.

   o Sodium: We should get no more than 1,500 milligrams per day, roughly equivalent to 2/3 teaspoon of table salt, for ages 19–50. From ages 51–70, 1,300 milligrams. Over age 70, 1,200 milligrams. No one should exceed 2,300 per day. Unfortunately, 95% of American men and 75% of American women exceed this amount. The major problem is with processed foods as many fast food products contain a whole day's intake.

   o Potassium: Our diets are deficient in potassium. High blood pressure is seen in industrialized countries due to diets low in potassium and high in sodium. In developing countries, the opposite is seen, with no high blood pressure. We need 4,700 milligrams per day, but most of us get less than half of that. Good sources are vegetables, especially leafy green ones, beans, and citrus fruits. Avoid taking supplements that provide too much as that can lead to abnormal heart rhythms.

❑ Sodium has been found to reduce bone density, which is a particular problem for women as we age.

Figure 16.14: Miscellaneous Vitamin and Mineral Facts

Useful Diet and Nutrition Resources

1. Activity Calorie Calculator
   http://www.primusweb.com/fitnesspartner/jumpsite/calculat.htm

2. American Association of Nutritional Sciences
   http://www.nutrition.org/

3. American Dietetic Association
   http://www.eatright.org/Public/

4. American Heart Association Food Pyramid
   http://www.deliciousdecisions.org/ee/afp.html

5. Dallas Dietetic Association Calorie Calculator
   http://www.dallasdietitian.com/calcalc.htm

6. Institute of Medicine—Created by the US government
   http://www.iom.edu/

7. Journal of the American College of Nutrition
   http://www.jacn.org/

Useful Diet and Nutrition Resources

8. Mayo Clinic Food and Nutrition Center
    Contains serving size guides, calorie counters, food pyramids, and special diets
    http://www.mayoclinic.com/findinformation/conditioncenters/centers.cfm?object id=000851DA-6222-1B37-8D7E80C8D77A0000

9. National Heart, Lung, and Blood Institute
    http://www.nhlbi.nih.gov/health
    BMI Calculator at http://nhlbisupport.com/bmi

10. Partnership for Essential Nutrition
    http://www.essentialnutrition.org/

11. University of Illinois Champaign/Urbana Nutrition Analysis Tool
    Analyze foods that you eat, including fast foods
    http://nat.crgq.com/index.html

12. US Department of Agriculture (USDA)

    ❑   Dietary Guidelines
        http://www.health.gov/dietaryguidelines/

    ❑   Dietary Guidelines 2005 (Proposed)
        http://www.health.gov/dietaryguidelines/dga2005/report/

    ❑   Food and Nutrition Information Center
        http://www.nal.usda.gov/fnic/etext/000108.html

    ❑   Interactive Healthy Eating Index
        Dietary assessment tool
        http://209.48.219.53/default.asp

    ❑   Nutrient Database Search
        http://www.nal.usda.gov/fnic/foodcomp/search/

    ❑   Nutritive Value of Foods
        Exhaustive list of foods and nutrient values
        http://www.nal.usda.gov/fnic/foodcomp/Data/HG72/hg72.html

Figure 16.15: Useful Diet and Nutrition Resources

Now that you have put together your healthy eating plan, let's move on to getting exercise, in Chapter 17.

Chapter

17

Exercise Daily

In this chapter we'll focus on why exercise is important, the types of exercise, and how to get exercise. By the end of this chapter you will have created your own exercise plan.

Why Exercise is Important

Exercise is not my favorite topic. To me, it's not a whole lot of fun. I've never really been athletic, and had no interest in playing sports. I'll admit it—it just never appealed to me. My Daddy taught me to play baseball, so I was able to, but I just never had a desire to go out for sports. But then, when I was in school, girls didn't play sports anyway. We were cheerleaders and majorettes, not jocks.

I've now accepted how important exercise is. It really is critical to our health. Not only does it strengthen your heart, it also helps you to avoid being overweight, dissipates stress, and increases your good cholesterol. Here are some other benefits:

- Reduced risk of heart disease: The Centers for Disease Control studied more than 13,000 people and found that getting vigorous exercise three times per week cut heart disease risk in half. Some new research also reported that our hearts stiffen up when we don't work them, and that seniors who are athletic have hearts that look and work just like those of younger folks.

- Reduced risk of breast cancer: Moderate levels of exercise reduce breast cancer in post-menopausal women.

- Reduced hot flashes: Women who are physically active experience fewer and less intense hot flashes, though extreme exercise can cause increased hot flashes. The key is to maintain a consistent level of exercise.

- Improved sleep: Post-menopausal women who exercise every day experience improved sleep, and those who exercise in the morning experience more benefit than those who exercise at night.

Types of Exercise

There are two major types of exercise programs for your heart – cardiovascular exercise and strength training.

1) **Cardiovascular exercise** builds your heart. A brisk 30–60 minute walk five or more times a week gets your heart pumping, burns calories, makes you feel better, and increases good cholesterol. You can do the same thing with a swim, run, or cardio workout. It's also an opportunity to think and de-stress, doubling your benefits. A heart rate monitor will help you stay within your heart's optimal range. The hardest part is shoehorning it into an already full schedule. When I don't have time to walk, I do it anyway. I'm more productive as a result, easily making up the time invested. I can't afford not to.

2) **Strength training** burns calories and builds muscle. Strength training, whether with free weights, weight machines, or resistance bands, is particularly valuable for women, burning about 200 calories for every 30 minutes and decreasing blood pressure and cholesterol. It also builds muscle, which burns more calories than fat, and boosts bone density, which is especially important following menopause to help avoid osteoporosis. Can you fit in strength training for 15–20 minutes two or three times a week in addition to your walking? If so, that's enough to keep you fit and healthy.

Getting Exercise

Many of you already have this one under control—congratulations! My hat's off to you. You work out, have personal trainers, do sports, or run.

Before my surgery, I didn't have it under control. Though I was getting some exercise, it just wasn't focused enough and consistent. My doctor made me give up running after a back injury years ago, and it was hard to work out when on the road. My job and travel were so time-consuming that it was hard to do anything more than grab snippets of time to walk. I just couldn't squeeze in an hour for driving round trip to the gym, and could rarely find time for my stair-stepper at home. On the road, entertaining customers left no time to exercise. Besides, I'd have been mortified if my customers had seen me looking like a "sweat hog" in the hotel gym. Can you relate to that? Are you concerned about who will see you at the gym?

When I left the hospital, my cardiologist insisted that I increase my exercise level. He told me to take a brisk walk every day—no less than 30 minutes, but with 60 minutes preferred. Some doctors recommend that you can get your exercise in increments, such as with three 10-minute sessions each day. My doctor said that you don't really get the HDL increase until you exceed thirty minutes. Obviously, we don't have exact answers.

Since my surgery, I've more than doubled my exercise, losing weight and burning off stress. I do a brisk 30–60 minute walk every day, and gym workouts when possible.

What about you? Do you focus every day on getting some vigorous cardiovascular activity (i.e., brisk walking, jogging, swimming, or working on cardio-workout equipment) to increase your heart rate and breathing rates? You can supplement that with mild activities (i.e., walking, housework, gardening, exercise, or yoga). Of course, strength training is a must. Before starting any exercise program, discuss it with your doctor.

Do you travel a lot? If so, how can you get exercise on the road?

1) When the weather is good, you can walk outside. When it's not, or you don't feel safe, you can walk in malls, airports, convention centers, and even the hotel. In my traveling to San Jose on business, I got to know just about every nook and cranny of the Westin Santa Clara and the adjoining Santa Clara Convention Center. Watching the conference activities going on each day at the convention center kept my walks interesting.

2) You can also work out in the hotel gym, if there is one. Of course, there are a lot of reasons to prefer doing workouts in your room, not the least of which is safety. Consider taking your workout gear with you—pack bands, plastic hand weights that you fill with water, and CDs or printouts of workout routines. Karen Hiser's Healthy Travel Network offers The Travel Fit Kit, which features resistance bands, a customizable exercise program CD, and a travel pouch for $19.95. You can also get a Hotel Room Workout on a laminated reference card for $5. Also check out her directory and reviews of hotel workout facilities. (See Appendix B for the link to her site.

Create Your Exercise Plan

To create your exercise plan, take a few minutes to think about the following questions and to write your answers in Figure 17.1, below.

1) What is my current exercise program like? How is it working for me?

2) What is my goal, what do I hope to accomplish, or how will I benefit?

3) What are my options for accomplishing my exercise goals, and what are the pros and cons of each?

4) What kind of exercise plan can I commit to? What will I do, and when will I do it? What is required (equipment, classes, gym membership, etc.) in order to accomplish it? What steps and interim stages will I commit to?

5) How will I know that I'm successful?

Exercise Goals

1. What is my current exercise program like? How is it working for me?

2. What is my goal, what do I hope to accomplish, or how will I benefit?

3. What are my options for accomplishing my exercise goals, and what are the pros and cons of each?

4. What kind of exercise plan can I commit to? What will I do, and when will I do it? What is required (equipment, classes, gym membership, etc.) in order to accomplish it? What steps and interim stages will I commit to?

5. How will I know that I'm successful?

Figure 17.1: Your Exercise Goals

From your answers in Figure 17.1, you can formulate your exercise plan, for which you'll use Figure 17.3. In Figure 17.2 is a sample to give you ideas for your exercise plan.

Exercise Plan and Targets

Exercise Program	Current	Ideal	Commitments/ Action Steps	Target Dates
Brisk walking	10 min/day	60 min/day	Start tomorrow	1 month
Weight training	Infrequent	3x/week	Enroll in gym	2 weeks
Cardio workout	Infrequent	3x/week	Enroll in gym	2 weeks
Yoga	None	1x/week	Find class and signup	1 month

Figure 17.2: Sample Exercise Plan and Targets

Now, in Figure 17.3, use your answers from Figure 17.1 to formulate your own personal exercise plan.

The Activity Calorie Calculator may be helpful in creating your plan as it calculates how many calories you'll burn for different activities and for different lengths of time (http://www.primusweb.com/fitnesspartner/jumpsite/calculat.htm).

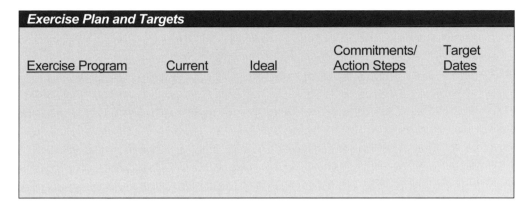

Figure 17.3: Your Exercise Plan and Targets

Now that you have done your exercise plan, let's focus on your attitude about stress and your stress plan, in Chapter 18.

A healthy attitude is contagious but don't wait to catch it from others.
Be a carrier.
Anonymous

Chapter

18

Attitude About Stress: How You Can Learn to Love Stress

In this chapter we will explore the impact of stress on our health, what causes us stress, what it does to us, and how to deal with it. By the end of this chapter you will have put together a plan for managing your stress.

The Impact of Stress

Is your life stressful? Whose isn't? Is the pace of your life too fast? Does it continue to get faster each year? Our speed-obsession is a major cause of our stress problem. For many of us, life seems to be spiraling out of control and stress is reaching epidemic proportions.

The reason stress is a problem is that it produces illness. It causes physical ailments, such as headaches and backaches, morale issues, decreased productivity, family issues, financial problems, substance abuse, and diminished quality of life. It also shuts down the immune system, causing such chronic diseases as heart disease, cancer, diabetes, and immune system disorders. These are the body's SOS signals of distress. Listen up.

Here are some startling personal and business statistics about stress-related illness.

- Fifty-two per cent of executives will die of stress-related illnesses, according to the Cooper Clinic.

- Eighty-five per cent of doctor visits are stress-related.

- Medical costs for those who are stressed are estimated at fifty per cent higher than for others.

- On-the-job stress accounts for up to forty per cent of employee turnover, and is the culprit in more than half of lost workdays as employees resort to taking "mental health days."

- US government figures indicate that stress-related illnesses cost us $26 billion in medical and disability costs and $95 billion in lost productivity each year.

- White-collar workers account for two-thirds of occupational stress, stress so severe that it causes significant time away from work, with almost half being away from work 31 days or more.

- In the two months following September 11, some New York hospitals saw heart attacks increase by as much as one-third and irregular heart rhythms increase by forty per cent, most likely brought on by physical and mental stress.

How did things get so bad? Where did this stress problem come from? I think it stemmed from *Internet time*. Do you remember that? That was where one Internet year equaled two months? When the dot-com bubble burst, some businesses breathed a sigh of relief and slowed down, but others continued their inexorable march and the ones that slowed down are now in catch-up mode. As we're pulling out of the tech slowdown, companies are revving back up to warp speed again.

You may be thinking that this impact on business doesn't impact you personally, and perhaps it doesn't directly, but with companies deferring hiring because healthcare costs for new employees are too burdensome, job creation lags and existing employees get more overburdened. Speed, and our stressed lifestyles, seriously affect us all and our economies.

What does stress do to you personally? When you get stressed, do you feel depressed? Do you get stomach upsets or ulcers? Do you get short-tempered and snap at people? Do you want to eat? Most people get one, or all, of these responses. Why does stress do this to us?

Stress causes biochemical responses in the body that date back to the caveman's "fight or flight" response. When cavemen were threatened by dangerous animals, cortisol, the stress hormone, shut down non-vital systems, such as digestion and the immune system, and diverted sugar to the muscles for fleeing. Today, though we're no longer threatened by dangerous animals, workplace and family stresses cause our bodies to respond much the same way. This puts us at risk for ulcers, colds, diabetes, cancer, and heart disease.

If stress were short-lived, like in caveman days, it wouldn't be so bad, but it's now persistent and pernicious. Our bodies short-circuit from a near-constant stress load that overworks the heart and upsets the body's normal insulin response. Cortisol slows down the metabolism to help you store up fat for energy and makes you gain weight. You crave cheeseburgers, fries, and other fattening foods, and once you've stored up fat for energy, cortisol won't let you waste that energy on needless exercise. **If you're dieting and exercising, but still not losing weight, do something about your stress.**

Some medical researchers postulate that it's actually anger in response to stress that causes most of our risk. They suggest that anger causes atrial fibrillation, a problem with the heart's rhythm, and churns out stress hormones that constrict blood vessels and increase blood pressure. Constricting of blood vessels can rupture plaques in the arteries, forming blood clots that block the arteries and cause heart attacks. Harvard researchers concluded that two per cent of heart attacks and strokes are brought on by anger, and men with anger and hostility are up to 30% more likely to experience atrial fibrillation. This effect was not observed among women, but that could change as women's stress loads more closely mirror those of men.

Stress can happen to any of us, including you! All it takes is a lifetime of eating things that accumulate in your blood vessels, followed by one stressful or frustrating incident, and that's it. That's why stressed lifestyles are such a risk, but you can eliminate much of your stress, and control most of it. We'll talk about that shortly.

Sources of Stress

What stresses you out? Let's start examining stress by looking at what are some things that cause women to be stressed. Work, for one.

People who work sitting down have more stress
than people who work standing up.
Mellanie True Hills

Job Demands and Uncertainty

The results of a recent USA TODAY survey into the causes of stress at work are shown in Figure 18.1. More than half of respondents cited the demands of the job as their primary source of stress. Others cited co-workers, bosses, and the fear of layoffs as top stressors.

Top Four Causes of Stress at Work	
Cause	Per Cent Citing
Job demands	54%
Co-workers	20%
Boss	10%
Fear of layoffs	8%

Figure 18.1: Top Four Causes of Stress at Work, Source: USA TODAY

On-the-job stress is one of the most pernicious sources of stress today, whether you're in an office, plant, or on the go.

Does your job cause you stress? Perhaps it's due to time pressures and too much to do at work. Many of us work in a 24x7, do it now, do more and more with less and less kind of world where the treadmill just goes faster and faster. Or maybe it's due to the economic uncertainties that just won't seem to go away, or the continued outsourcing of jobs offshore. Perhaps you are afraid of what may happen to your job, especially if you've seen others around you affected. Many of us have just come to accept constantly spiraling job demands as being better than the alternatives.

Do you remember that old "I Love Lucy" episode where she and Ethel worked in the candy factory? The candy just kept coming, faster and faster, so to keep up, Lucy crammed candy into her mouth until she was overwhelmed. Do you ever feel overwhelmed like that at work as you just can't stop the work from coming at you? That's probably why so many of us work through lunch—we just can't keep up.

Do you have to multitask at work? Is everything a #1 priority? Are you overwhelmed with too much information? Do interruptions interrupt the interruptions? Is every day like that for you? It's gotten really crazy! It's hard not to get stressed!

My life was like that. I had an always-on, 24x7, high-tech, road-warrior life. As I've mentioned, I worked almost around the clock as it was difficult to keep up with the productivity treadmill and the information wave that constantly threatened to push me under. Constant pressure to overdeliver on seemingly impossible objectives led to rampant overscheduling and multitasking in an attempt to keep up. It became impossible to focus on a single thing at a time due to all the competing demands.

That's not an unusual story today—most of you probably relate to it, and many of you are living that same story. Unrelenting job demands cause us to do crazy things, like conference calls or returning voicemails every time we get behind the wheel, or to work at airports and on the plane no matter how exhausted or sleep deprived we are from traveling. We leave voicemails until the plane door closes, and the moment the flight arrives we start checking voicemails, pagers, and e-mail.

I've seen this kind of intense time pressure lead to quirky, and even questionable, behavior, such as trying to negotiate the airport security gauntlet while on conference calls, making cell phone calls from airplanes when all electronic devices are supposed to be turned off, or worst of all, making phone calls from the restroom. I've known several colleagues over the years that have had to replace phones that got submerged in the restroom. (Interestingly, none were women.)

This kind of multitasking is not only counterproductive, as studies have shown, but also leads to health issues as the adrenalin in the body continues to build with little opportunity to dissipate during the day. Multitasking, fast-talking, over-committed, always-in-a-hurry adrenaline junkies may be driving themselves to heart attacks. You probably see lots of them around you, and may even be one yourself. You know who you are. We Type A's create stress for ourselves, and sometimes for others.

Another cause of stress at work can come from being in a job for which you aren't a good fit. Have you ever done such a good job that you got a promotion to the next level, only to find out that you weren't happy in the new situation? Maybe you're an individual contributor and discovered that you didn't like management. Or perhaps you were so good in an operational position that you were asked to work as a liaison between information technology and the business. Maybe you're good with customers and loved your customer support role, and now are in a role that involves selling to those same customers. Job-fit issues can lead to stress.

Disparities in team contribution can be another cause of stress. A friend recently commented on what she saw as women's greater sense of responsibility for team results, at least in her industry. She felt that some men get appointed to teams and just blow it off, whereas women tend to feel personally responsible for team results and may carry a disproportionate share of the team load. In that case, team commitments become another work-related stressor.

Stress in the workplace continues to grow. Between the threat of layoffs and downsizing, doing more with less, and the recovery that never seems to quite take hold, employees just can't keep up and many are near burnout. This will become a costly problem for companies as numerous studies have shown that increased stress in the workplace coupled with increased job demands is negatively impacting employee's mental and physical health. Up to one-third of employees suffer from stress-related illnesses, driving up health care costs and driving down company productivity. In addition, stress from job insecurity also contributes to increased workplace accidents, up to an 80% increase, and increased workplace violence. Thus it behooves companies to tackle head-on the issues causing stress in the workplace.

People forget how fast you did a job – but
they remember how well you did it.
Howard Newton

Information Overload

Another source of stress on the job is information overload. Is that an issue for you? I used to be so inundated with informational e-mails in a previous job that a lot just got deleted unread. My boss at the time, knowing that we were all overwhelmed, told us just to delete a lot of our e-mails without reading them. When we joked that we'd start with his e-mails, he didn't think that was funny—no sense of humor!

A lot of people are addicted to e-mail. Are you? When your e-mail icon pops up, do you just have to check it? Do you get up in the middle of the night and check e-mail before going back to bed?

In some high-tech companies, e-mail was the last thing you did before leaving the office and the first thing you did when you got home, even before kissing your spouse! The norm regarding e-mail stems from the way company executives handle it. I once had a boss that would never send e-mail during the day as he was in meetings all day, but he would pummel us with nightly e-mails until 1AM and again starting at 4 AM. That set a tone that employees were expected to reply to e-mails all evening and before the workday began. That boss was only responding to the actions of other executives up the line. Company e-mail practices and expectations come from the top. If you're in a top position at your company, what messages are you sending your employees?

Top executives' practices also dictate whether the organization is an e-mail culture or a voice-mail one. Heaven help you if you're an e-mail person in a voice-mail culture, or vice versa. That's a stressor.

Figure 18.2 contains some lessons I learned about stress from dealing with my e-mail while writing this book.

Life Lessons From E-mail

I'm back from four weeks of travel in the RV with my family, which took us to National Parks across Arizona, Nevada, Utah, New Mexico, and Texas.

During the business part of the trip, I had planned to keep up with my e-mail, but that proved to be quite a challenge. I'm not an e-mail newbie, having managed an early IBM-mainframe-based e-mail system for a large manufacturer almost two decades ago and led JCPenney's Internet project in the early 1990s, but even so, this time e-mail proved to be much more than I bargained for.

What we envisioned way back then for e-mail has come, and gone. It's now a big pain due to the overwhelming quantities of junk mail. E-mail has become totally unreliable. In fact, Information Week magazine found that only 60–70% of e-mail reaches the intended recipient. You're not getting 30–40% of your e-mail, and it's not all junk that is getting weeded out—you may be missing important e-mails, too.

Have you ever re-sent e-mail, asking "Did you get this?" Or do you ever call to make sure your message survived the e-mail gauntlet? Of course. How ridiculous is what we've had to resort to!

I knew that on the trip some RV parks would have WiFi or instant-on phones, but most would not, so keeping up with e-mail might be a challenge. After all, when you're in a 36-foot motorhome with a "toad" (RV-speak for towed car), you can't just swing into the

Life Lessons From E-mail

nearest Starbucks to connect up and take a hit of e-mail. And, as hard as it is to believe, you can travel clear across West Texas, for 600 miles, and never see a single Starbucks (or Wal-mart either, for that matter). Thankfully, the state of Texas is putting wireless into rest areas soon to encourage drowsy drivers to take a break.

Maybe getting e-mail wouldn't be such a big challenge after all—a WiFi network has sprung up connecting truck stops across the country as truckers need frequent access to e-mail and corporate intranets. I signed up, and could just see myself downloading e-mail at warp speed while my husband fueled the RV. Thank goodness for technology!

A few days into the trip, it was time to check it out. My computer easily latched onto the wireless network, so I signed on and was ready to fly. Web at high speed. Yes!

But I couldn't access e-mail. Between deleting cookies, closing the spyware checker, adjusting Internet security, and changing the firewall, something worked. Pulling message 1 of 2,958.

Then the wireless connection dropped. I tried again, and e-mail started over. Why couldn't it start where it left off? After a few more dropped connections, I packed it in, presuming a problem at this location.

Next truck stop, same story. Pulling 1 of 4,796 messages. Then the e-mail software blew up! I'd packed archival backups, but didn't think to bring the software installation disk. Plan B—by dial-up at the next RV park, I traded up to more cooperative e-mail software.

Even with the new software, there were conflicts between e-mail and the WiFi network. I'm not a WiFi newbie, but couldn't get them to work together, and somewhere along the way, my new e-mail Inbox and Sent messages vaporized. OK, it's time to start vacation and forget about this infernal e-mail.

When I returned home, my e-mail provider rebuilt the corrupted e-mail indexes and got me back in business.

You're wondering why I didn't let the system filter all that junk. Fair enough. Unfortunately, generic junk filtering doesn't work well for health topics, throwing away too much good mail and keeping the bad. That's why I love my Bayesian filter that learns my criteria, but requires downloading all messages, which usually isn't a problem.

What are some life lessons from this e-mail adventure?

1. E-mail and technology can bring stress into our lives, causing us to feel out of control. Just accept it and move on.
2. We all feel out of control at times, and can empathize with others when they do.
3. Stay productive. When something isn't working, let it go.
4. Reach out to others for help. My husband found me a new e-mail tool.
5. When my Inbox vaporized, I had a profound sense of relief as I couldn't do anything about it. I let it go and enjoyed my vacation.
6. I came back refreshed, rejuvenated, re-energized, and revitalized—even ready to tackle e-mail!

Figure 18.2: Life Lessons From E-mail

Co-workers and Bosses

We've all experienced difficult co-workers, and perhaps even a toxic boss or two. Though you've probably had some wonderful bosses and co-workers, you have probably also had your share of ineffectual ones. We all have.

One stressor in the workplace is rudeness and lack of civility. Actually, it's not just in the workplace—it's been in politics lately, too, as the language in political campaigns has gotten far more colorful than usual. The problem is just getting worse in the workplace as some employees have come to feel that it is perfectly acceptable to be rude and disruptive in the name of getting the job done, and because they are entitled to.

An insensitive boss is another stressor. I know someone who was off for surgery whose boss called just after the surgery to grill her about plans for returning to work. It later became obvious that the boss had paperwork to fill out and needed to check it off the to-do list.

We're not all alike, so people with a different workstyle can cause us stress at work. I have noticed a phenomenon that I call *Being a Night Person in a Morning Person Company*. Figure 18.3 explores some differences between morning people and night people.

Differences Between Morning People and Night People	
Morning People	Night People
Consider a seven o'clock meeting to be the second or third meeting of the morning.	Consider a seven o'clock meeting to be dinner
Hit the deck running	Hit the snooze button
Want to beat the morning rush hour	What morning rush hour? They're still asleep.
Are most productive from 6AM to 12 noon	Are also most productive from 6–12, PM that is
For a 10AM meeting in another city they take the 6AM flight	For a 10AM meeting in another city they take the late flight the night before
Think morning people are industrious, creative, and bright, but think that night people are lazy, undisciplined, and slow	Think night people are industrious, creative, and bright, but think that morning people are on drugs
Tend toward sales, marketing, manufacturing, and customer support jobs	Tend toward engineering and programming jobs (no wonder tech firms have culture clashes)

Figure 18.3: Differences Between Morning People and Night People

Neither type is right or wrong, but these differences do cause culture clashes within companies, and therefore stress. If you're a morning person, what do you think when a night person comes rolling in at 8:30 or later? Does it drive you crazy? It often does.

In one of my jobs, my team had lots of night people, as tech folks often are. While it didn't bother me when they weren't in early, it drove some of my peers crazy. Yet my team's output was staggering. They were **adults**—I let them work when, where, and how they were most productive.

A couple of other stressors in the workplace are internal competition and, my personal favorite, obsessing over unimportant tasks that don't benefit customers or stakeholders.

Commute and Traffic

In some cities, the commuting traffic can be horrendous. A scary study by the Texas Transportation Institute found that drivers in one-third of cities spend at least half as much time stuck in traffic each year as they do on vacation. And here in Austin, we have been having spots on morning TV encouraging drivers to drive less aggressively when they hit the freeways in the morning. Isn't that amazing!

Travel

Does travel cause you stress? This is a commonly listed stressor since September 11. Are you more afraid now? More stressed?

Air travel is no longer a luxury, and business travel is especially stressful, particularly having to unpack all electronic gear and disrobe to go through security. Is it second nature now to remove your belt, jacket, jewelry, and shoes? Or do you have a metal-free travel outfit to help you breeze through security? That's what I used to do. I also kept my jewelry packed and put it on after clearing security. We've mostly gotten used to dealing with airport security, even though the rules vary from one airport to the next, and from one day to the next.

How does it make you feel when you go through security and get picked for extra screening? I don't like being patted down—it's intrusive to be touched in such private places, and is only getting worse. We've had to accept it and learn to live with it—if you're traveling by air, you must endure it.

What really bugs me about airport security is having someone totally unpack my luggage for random screening and hand it back in such disarray that I have to start over and repack it. Even worse, though maybe this is extra picky, I can't help thinking about how many other bags screeners have touched and wondering what germs they are leaving on my stuff. I resent having everything in the toiletries bag pulled out, and them touching my toothbrush and clean underwear even though I've packed them in see-thru bags. It's crazy—what kind of weapon could I really be hiding in a bra or a toothbrush anyway?

Some times you breeze right through, and other times you're picked for extra screening on every leg of the trip. Some of it makes no sense. Let's say you bought a round-trip ticket on a single airline, and when you got to the airport you discovered that one leg is flown by a code-share partner. The system designers treated that single ticket as multiple one-ways, flagging you for extra screening on every leg. How crazy is that?

Why do they pull us aside for tweezers and eyelash curlers and yet let pocket knives and corkscrews sail right through? Recently, a guy mistakenly left a corkscrew in his toiletry kit following a driving trip. The Transportation Security Agency (TSA) agent consulted with his supervisor, who decided to let him keep the corkscrew. When told that the traveler was a volunteer law officer, the TSA agent allowed that if he had known he wouldn't have bothered to ask his supervisor. This reminds me of the old "Airplane" movie—they stopped Grandma, but let the guerillas through carrying massive weapons. Don't you just love it when Grandma absent-mindedly wanders off while waiting to have her knitting needles inspected and when TSA can't find her they close the airport and make everyone be re-screened. Ah, life imitating art, post-9/11-style!

Most ridiculous of all is the detailed inspection of pilots. Do they think that the pilots might hijack a plane? Aren't those the guys and gals we're already entrusting with our lives each time we get on board? How ridiculous is that? And yet, they let airport cleaning crews and vendors through virtually unscreened.

If you travel multiple times a week, as I did, you get used to it and take steps to minimize the impact, but you still don't have to like it. You can control some of the frustration, but it still affects you in subtle ways. As a road warrior, I learned many tricks to minimize frustration, but they don't work every time.

Another travel stressor is food. September 11 provided most airlines the excuse to cut out meals, at least from flights under 4–5 hours. From Austin, we just don't get meals going anywhere. Have you resorted to carrying your own brown bag, or do you seek healthy food at airports? Healthy airport food—that seems like such an oxymoron for most airports. Taking frequent trips across time zones means that you must factor in what to do about meals on each leg of the trip—like there's not enough other stuff to deal with on the road already.

It's not just the flights that make travel stressful. How about getting enough sleep on trips? You get into a hotel late, still keyed up from travel, and can't sleep. Maybe it's a horrendous bed, or noise coming through paper-thin walls, or rooms that are just plain filthy or buggy, like when I found a dead scorpion under my pillow one night and wondered if there were lives ones still hiding in my room. If you've traveled much, you have encountered all of these, and more.

Since travel is stressful, and can put our health at risk, I can just see it now—a rash of lawsuits against the TSA and the airlines for stress-induced wrongful death!

Personal Relationships

Other people, and their habits, can drive us crazy. If you're married or in a relationship, did you notice when that relationship first started that sometimes little things got on your nerves? Was it the tube of toothpaste—rolled or flattened? Or was it the toilet paper—over or under? Or the toilet seat—up or down? Maybe it was the TV remote, with one of you being a "channel flipper".

When my husband and I first married (that's been a while—today is our thirty-second wedding anniversary), we figured that none of that was worth stressing over. We accepted each other's differences and moved on to the more important things in life. When those differences surface, we look for stress-free solutions. We're currently re-doing my home office, so I work temporarily in the dining room. My husband monitors news, business, and weather throughout the day, which I sometimes hear in my makeshift office. Turning the TV on and off stresses components (he's an electrical engineer) so when he leaves the room he mutes the TV. Sometimes he gets busy or distracted, so one day as I searched for the remote, I decided to create a subtle reminder. I folded a neon sheet of paper into a tent card, wrote "Did I mute the TV?" on it, and placed it on the landing as a gentle reminder for when he heads upstairs to his office. Most little things like that aren't worth stressing over.

Children

Do your kids cause you stress? Is it the terrible twos? Or a teenager that just turned into an alien? As a colleague used to say, "Sixteen is the terrible-twos times eight, with a driver's license." I'll bet that's comforting to those of you facing the teen years. I'm assured, however, by friends that teens really do get their brains back some time in their early twenties.

Do you have dogs as well as kids? Which is better behaved? Let me guess—is it the dog? When we tell our golden retriever, Sandy, to sit, stop, wait, or any other command, she obeys. When we tell her "night, night," she goes straight upstairs and puts herself to bed. How well does that work with kids? Do you ever wish you could send the kids to obedience school?

Perhaps your stress comes from the kids' relentless schedule of activities—soccer, baseball, T-ball, basketball, music lessons, karate, Scouts, camp, etc. Do you run straight from work to their games or practices? Is rush hour the calm between the storms? (I used to have a cartoon that said "Ah, what a relief—rush hour traffic!") Do you have to resort to drive-by fast food, which is now a major contributor to obesity in kids and adults?

What about day care challenges, including summer breaks and sick kids? Do you flip a coin with your spouse to see who stays home, or do you work out all kinds of tortuous arrangements, such as one working in the morning and the other in the afternoon, or juggling meetings to cover?

Parents

More and more of us are becoming "the sandwich generation," being squeezed by the challenges of simultaneously caretaking for both our kids and our parents. Parenting our parents also makes us confront our own fears about aging. My friend, Jim Comer, wrote a wonderful book, Parenting Your Parents, available at http://www.ParentingYourParents.com, which may help those of you facing this challenge.

Triple Threat

Women (and some men) are dealing with juggling the triple threat—balancing job, marriage or relationship (and sex), and kids, along with everything else. Women tend to be natural nurturers, carrying the load of supporting the emotional needs of family, colleagues, and friends. Often, we're so busy with family, career, faith, volunteering, social life, and meeting the needs of others that finding balance and meeting our own needs seems impossible. Work invades our personal lives, leading to blending and multitasking rather than balance. Blending and integrating all of our roles is fine as long as we don't let it squeeze out taking time for **us**.

What about the "quality time" conundrum that we women often face? After being squeezed all day at work, do you try to shoehorn in quality time with your family at night while juggling homework, school projects, school events, church, sports, and other events?

Does guilt over all the roles you are juggling cause you stress? Do you feel guilt at work because you're not at home, or guilt at home because you have work that you need to do? For many years, there was tension between the career moms and the stay-at-home moms, with both feeling guilty. What are your subconscious messages telling you? Are those messages positive or negative? Subconscious guilt messages can be thought of as *brain spam*—we need to filter them out so they don't clog our brains or stress us out.

Of course, certain times of the year are more stressful, too. The extra load from starting back to school or the holidays may cause you to go over the cliff.

Financial or Retirement Concerns

When the dot-com bubble burst, many who had planned to retire early gave up those plans. And for many of us, there is insecurity as to whether our jobs will continue to exist, especially in light of the many jobs being sent overseas. That squeezes our personal lives due to more and more concern about whether we can afford not to work the outrageous hours and whether we can take time off for vacation, never mind whether we can even afford it since we haven't had raises in years.

Health

One final area of stress is our health, and that of our families. For example, do you get stressed at certain times of the month? Of course.

Since women tend to manage the health of the family, it is often hard to find the time to take care of our own health. When you notice a change in your health, do you get stressed trying to figure out whether to see the doctor for it, and how to shoehorn it into everything else you do?

It's even worse for those without health insurance, which is a national crisis in the US. More than forty million Americans don't have health insurance, so for most uninsured the emergency room is the primary care provider.

Now that we've looked at some of the sources of stress, let's move on to looking at how to overcome those stresses.

How Do You Deal With Your Stress?

Stress is largely within our control. It's actually the symptom, not the disease, and is the product of a number of factors, such as lack of sleep, improper diet, or insufficient exercise, making it difficult for us to deal with the curves that life throws us.

Most of us know how to deal with stress, but it's hard to focus when you're in the midst of it. You're just too close to it. My goal in this section is to remind you of some steps you can take to deal with stress, and to give you some ideas that you may not think about when you are stressed. The best thing you can do in the middle of a stressful event is to stand back and view it objectively, but that's hard.

Perspective: Control Your Emotions

The most important thing in dealing with your stress is your attitude about it. It's not what happens to you, it's how you handle it. While exercise dissipates stress, a positive attitude lets you turn bad stress into good so that it doesn't overwhelm you. I hope you'll chose to roll with the punches and view your stresses positively.

Start by using some techniques to calm yourself until you can deal with the stress rationally. Take time out with deep breathing or a walk around the block. Stress increases blood pressure, so deep breathing helps relax the blood vessels. Or find a way to lighten up and laugh. When you're calmed down, you can flip things around to look at them positively or from the other person's perspective. Studies have shown that such techniques can significantly lower blood pressure. The _Relieve Stress_ program that I mentioned in Chapter 16 may help reduce your stress—see Appendix B for how to get it.

Sometimes life has a way of teaching us what we need. As I was working on this chapter, something stressful happened, and I knew that I had to get focused again. I sat down on the floor and started brushing our golden retriever. She was ready for her afternoon nap and seemed to be saying "OK, Mom, you can brush me as long as you don't mind me napping while you're doing it." With each stroke of the brush, my stress diminished, and when we were done, she snuggled in my lap to say thanks. Within ten minutes I was back at work and my effectiveness had increased significantly.

Another way to deal with stress is to look at things differently. For example, have you ever awakened late the morning of a big meeting, and in a panic, thrown on your makeup and clothes, sped to work, fought traffic, whipped into Starbucks for your coffee fix, spilled your coffee on yourself, and arrived late for the meeting only to discover that you were expected to make a presentation? Talk about stressful, or is it? If you can perceive it as not being stressful, and just go with the flow, you'll be much healthier.

Sometimes, something that seems bad could actually be good if you looked at it differently. Are you old enough to remember the movie, Pollyanna? Pollyanna was a young girl who saw something good in everything around her, even the bad things. It may sound corny, but a Pollyanna attitude is much healthier and easier than letting things eat at you.

Your perspective on stress, and on life in general, can make a big difference in your longevity as pointed out by a number of studies. Some examples include:

- Several studies have shown that women with depression symptoms have up to a 50% greater risk of dying from heart attack, and those who have both heart disease and depression have a 45% greater risk of stroke.

- A study reported in the _Mayo Clinic Proceedings_ (http://www.mayoclinic.com/invoke.cfm?id=MC00014) in August of 2002 found that optimistic people had a 50 per cent lower risk of premature death than pessimists. Optimists were also happier, calmer, and experienced greater energy levels, confirming that the mind and body really are linked.

- A report in the *Journal of Personality and Social Psychology* (http://www.apa.org/journals/psp.html) in August of 2002 indicated that older individuals who viewed aging optimistically lived 7.5 years longer than those with a pessimistic attitude about aging.

Optimism is not only important for dealing with stress, it can also extend your longevity.

Optimists roll with the punches, which I learned even more about on our stress-reducing girl's getaway to Italy. While we were in Rome, the European Union leaders met (they stayed at our hotel), and there were violent demonstrations, closing downtown to vehicle traffic. We avoided the morning protests, but the afternoon was my sister's last chance to visit a designer boutique in Rome that was similar to hers. It just happened to be one block from the demonstrations.

When we left the shop and headed for the subway, we found ourselves marching in the midst of labor demonstrators who were headed off to party. As we all waited patiently on the subway platform, millions of us, the trains suddenly stopped. Our limited Italian didn't help us to understand the announcement, but a young Italian explained it to us—it was a sympathy work stoppage. Millions of us were now stranded, with no cars or taxis in the city, and it was getting dark. Our new friend, Paolo, was headed to the same station, so together we plotted a bus route.

Surprisingly, there was no anger or frustration in the crowd—the Italians just took it in stride. If that had occurred in other places, such as the US, tempers might have flared. Fortunately, as we started to leave the station, the subways resumed and we headed for our hotel.

I've since learned that Italians have a much lower incidence of heart disease. Perhaps it's the Mediterranean Diet, of fish, vegetables, healthy tomatoes, pasta, and the good, Omega-3 fatty acids in olives and olive oil, or perhaps it's the wine. Or maybe it's their attitude, rolling with the punches, partying instead of stressing, and of course, working far fewer hours than us hard-charging Americans.

How can we adopt *that* kind of attitude? We can start by dealing with our stress one baby step at a time—find a single thing to think differently about, or to do something about. For example, if your boss, employee, or co-worker drives you crazy, can you adjust your attitude to relieve some of that stress? Or can you have a conversation with that person to deal with the problem? Is there something that you can get off your plate to relieve some of your stress? Is there something that you're responsible for, but that you can't control, and that you can shift responsibility for to those that do control it? At the very least, leave your stress at work, and don't take it home with you.

> *The last of the human freedoms is to choose one's attitudes.*
> Victor Frankl, 1905–1997, Holocaust Survivor and Author

> *If you don't like something, change it.*
> *If you can't change it, change your attitude.*
> Maya Angelou, 1928– , Author and Poet

Prioritize: How Does It Fit Your Plan?

Obviously, you can't do it all. There just isn't enough time. The next step is to sort out what is important and where to focus your energy so that you can get the right balance in your life. I learned a lesson about that while on vacation.

My husband, our teenage son, and I were in our RV driving toward Hoover Dam. The drive from Phoenix was long and arduous, with only construction stops to penetrate the boredom. The temperature had already passed 100 degrees when we left Phoenix early that morning, and had only worsened as we traversed the desert. The generator kept overheating, cutting off the air conditioning. It did so again in the blistering heat as the RV was inspected by Homeland Security so that we could cross the dam.

As we approached the dam, the view was extraordinary. My husband negotiated the tight switchbacks slowly, steadily, and intently. I was nervous just watching, but he skillfully maneuvered the massive 17–ton motorhome, which was 8 ½ feet wide and 52 feet long with car in tow, over the dam and through the tight turns without scraping rocks or oncoming vehicles.

What a relief when we reached the other side and started up the steep grade. My son resumed reading, and I checked the maps for our turn. Suddenly, a warning light pulsed a vivid red—ENGINE HOT. I noticed the outdoor temperature displayed on the dash—119 degrees.

My engineer husband sequenced through possible solutions for the diesel engine. Suddenly, he said, "Oh, yeah, downshift," as he slid the transmission into lower gear. Within minutes the engine returned to normal and we made it to Las Vegas that night.

Have you ever had a day like that—full of frustrations that made you feel like you were carrying a heavy load uphill and overheating? Next time, think "Oh, yeah, downshift," and drop into lower gear to relieve the strain.

I don't mean drop out—just take time to analyze, prioritize, simplify, change your view, slow down, or quit multitasking. When you get more and more work thrown at you, downshift. When your boss drives you crazy, downshift. When family challenges overwhelm you, downshift.

Interestingly, after being downshifted while going up that hill, the computerized transmission "learned," and as we started up the next hill, it downshifted automatically. Can you teach your body to do that automatically?

Downshift? Are you thinking, well how exactly do you do that? What do you mean? That's what I had to figure out when I left the hospital.

Having a life-changing experience altered my perspective. I knew that I had to do whatever it took to be there for my family. I had to prioritize and seize control of my work, travel, and life. As a Type A, off-the-scale driver, that's hard, but if I didn't I'd be back in the hospital for open-heart surgery. Managing my stress had finally become crucial.

Getting my work under control was a huge challenge. My colleagues and I worked long days and weekends, but that couldn't continue as my body had to heal. I limited myself to ten hour days and minimal weekends. I also traveled less frequently, and did more virtual meetings. When I did travel, I was less fanatical about working. I prioritized ruthlessly, eliminating anything that didn't meet my #1 priority, meeting customer needs.

Though I still do make phone calls when I'm in the car (hands-free, or course), I try to do calls that are more social and require less heavy-duty concentration. It's just too dangerous to do calls that require a lot of intense brainstorming and focus. Sometimes I just focus on letting my mind rest rather than making calls.

How can you deal with the productivity treadmill? One way is to align your goals with your organization's goals and your boss' goals. That lets you offload things that don't contribute. Prioritize – what is most important to you, and what can go by the wayside?

I recently had to make a tough priority decision. I was offered a volunteer position that I would have loved to take, but my volunteer plate was already full and I decided that I just had to pass for the time being. Maybe it's the right thing to do later, but for my health, now is not the time.

Other factors in the HEART Program—healthy eating, exercise, and rest and relaxation—help you deal with stress, too. While each is dealt with in depth in a separate chapter, I've included here some ideas related specifically to stress.

Healthy Eating (Chapter 16)

What we eat can be a major factor in how well we deal with stress. Brain chemicals, called neurotransmitters (i.e., adrenaline and serotonin), control brain function. Since they're made from the foods we eat, a poor diet impairs the body's ability to make these chemicals. Our bodies need proteins, fresh fruits and vegetables, grains, vitamins B and C, and magnesium, which are especially important in making the brain chemicals that help the body handle stress.

If you're feeling stressed, check whether you're eating properly. Are you living on high-fat and high-sugar junk and fast foods, or are you overdoing caffeine (coffee, tea, sodas, and chocolate)? Overloading the body with fats, refined sugars, and caffeine can throw it way out of balance.

Diet is especially important for us Type-A adrenaline junkies. High protein and caffeine-laden foods increase adrenaline, shoving the body into overdrive. Those who consistently use adrenaline at work keep their bodies in perpetual fight or flight mode, causing fat and sugar junk food cravings to build stores for the next emergency. Adrenaline also supercharges the heart, which is why we're starting to correlate high stress with heart disease. Pouring more and more adrenaline into an overstressed body is like pouring gasoline onto a fire, and in extreme cases can lead to fear, anxiety, and paranoia.

Keeping the adrenaline system constantly in overdrive also lowers the body's serotonin, a neurotransmitter that makes you feel good. By depressing serotonin levels, you may be at risk for anxiety and depression. Getting enough sleep (7–8 hours per night) rebuilds serotonin, as does eating turkey, bananas, walnuts, avocados, and tomatoes.

When you're under stress, a diet of vegetables and high-quality, low-fat protein can optimize the body to withstand stress. Everyone's body is different, so your nutritional needs may vary. Your doctor can advise you on the right diet for you, or perhaps direct you to a nutritionist who can.

If you feel stressed, take a moment to examine why and to identify what you can do immediately about it. Be sure that you are eating properly and getting enough rest.

Exercise (Chapter 17)

One way to dissipate stress is through exercise, which simulates the body fleeing from danger. That uses up the chemicals released into the bloodstream.

When you're exercising, avoid multitasking, another source of stress. Don't be tempted to listen to learning tapes or do conference calls. Just let your mind clear to de-stress, reflect, and meditate. Give your body a chance to replenish from the demands of multitasking at work and home.

Rest, Relaxation, and Rejuvenation (Chapter 19)

Sleep deprivation can seriously impair our ability to deal with stress, and even exacerbate the smallest stressors. Consider the poor woman who was recently at the center of a national security incident. She lost her father, had an operation, her husband lost his job, and then her brother was hospitalized, causing her to become exhausted from two sleepless nights. The following morning, while driving to pick up her mother-in-law from President Bush's speech, she drove past traffic barricades where police and Secret Service tried to stop her. She drove on, crashed into the civic center, and was pulled from the car kicking and fighting, landing in jail. Talk about having a bad day, all from stress-induced sleep deprivation.

Sleep deprivation may also have been the cause of a recent incident of spam rage. A Silicon Valley programmer allegedly threatened to torture and kill employees and executives at a direct-marketing company that he claimed was spamming him, even after being assured by the company president that the spams weren't from his company. The programmer, a survivor of testicular cancer, was frustrated by the barrage of e-mails promising male sex organ enhancement.

If you are getting enough sleep to help you stay in control, you're more likely to overlook the little things that could drive you crazy, or to deal with them diplomatically and in a non-personal, non-threatening, non-accusatory manner.

Another step is to slow down. I follow the ancient philosophy of **Go slow to get there fast**. If you get to moving too fast, you make mistakes and end up re-doing it. By doing it at a more conscious level you may actually get it done faster and avoid re-doing it. This applies especially to multitasking as studies have shown the fallacy of human multitasking. A study reported in the August 2001 issue of the Journal of Experimental Psychology (http://www.apa.org/journals/xhp/press_releases/august_2001/xhp274763.html) pointed out that each time you change tasks, the body takes a certain amount of time to get re-oriented to the new task. The most efficient way to work is a single-threaded approach of focusing on one thing at a time.

One of the ways I relax is with our golden retriever. She knows when I'm stressed, and nuzzles me to rub her. We go for long walks together to enjoy nature. To her, there are no strangers—only friends that she just hasn't yet met. I've learned a lot because when we walk, she stops and visits with everyone, and focuses on enjoying the trip rather than on reaching the destination.

Interests outside of job and family also provide necessary balance and can relieve stress. That might include a hobby, religion or faith, volunteering, or social activities. Research has found that those with friends and social connections have less risk of heart disease.

Once my lifestyle was under control, I knew it was time to give back. I volunteer with the American Heart Association as a speaker and fundraiser, and have just joined the local board of directors.

Create Your Plan to Deal with Stress

Now it's time to evaluate the stress in your life and to create a plan to deal with it. Let's first assess your stress level. On the stress meter below, in Figure 18.4, mark an X on the first line to show your stress level for work and an X on the second line to show your stress level in your personal life. Use a scale of 1–10, with 1 being low and 10 being high.

Personal Stress Profile
What's my work stress level?
1 (Low)   (High) 10
What's my personal stress level?
1 (Low)   (High) 10

Figure 18.4: Your Personal Stress Profile

Do you know what is causing your stress, and what impact it has on you? In Figure 18.5, you'll find a sample list of stressors and impacts that were listed by recent seminar attendees.

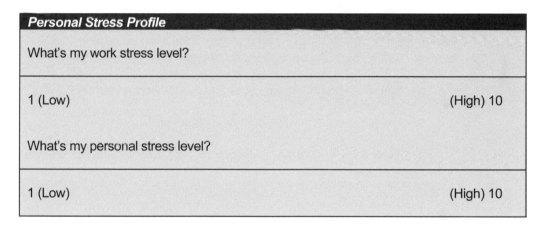

Stress Inventory	
Stressor	What It Does To Me
Job/boss	Frustration, headaches, dread, anger
Travel	Insomnia on the road
Too much to do	Frantic and short-tempered
Family conflict	Nervous and frazzled

Figure 18.5: Sample Stress Inventory

Now, do a quick inventory for you—what is stressing you and what impact does it have on you? Take a moment to fill in your own list, in Figure 18.6.

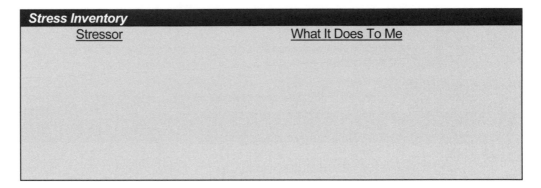

Figure 18.6: Your Personal Stress Inventory

What can you do about these stressors? In Figure 18.7, take the time to answer the following questions.

1)   What are the things that are causing me the most stress?

2)   What can I do to eliminate the stress or to change the way I respond to it?

3)   What benefits will I gain from these changes?

4)   What will I commit to changing in the next month? Next quarter? Next year?

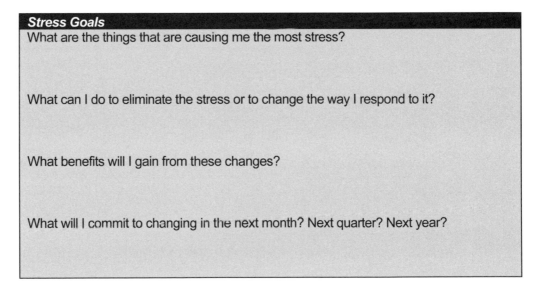

Figure 18.7: Your Personal Stress Goals

In Figure 18.8 is a sample stress plan. It was created based on the answers to the questions in Figure 18.7. In the sample, for each stressor listed, I identified the current and ideal situations as well as steps to bridge the gap and target dates for accomplishing the action steps.

Stress Plan/Targets				
Stressor	Current	Ideal	Commitments/ Action Steps	Target Dates
Job	Overwhelming job	Achieve balance	Discuss priorities with boss	Next week, in 1x1 with boss
Travel	Problems sleeping	Well rested	Travel early in day; Request hotel accommodation	Next trip, in 2 weeks
Work/life balance	Unbalanced life	Time for outside activities	Volunteer	One month

Figure 18.8: Sample Stress Plan and Targets

Now build your own stress plan using Figure 18.9. Use your answers from Figure 18.7 to identify areas to address, along with the current and ideal states, your committed steps, and target dates.

Stress Plan/Targets				
Stressor	Current	Ideal	Commitments/ Action Steps	Target Dates

Figure 18.9: Your Stress Plan and Targets

Now that you've built your stress plan, let's move on to rest, relaxation, and rejuvenation, in Chapter 19.

Half our life is spent trying to find something to do
with the time we have rushed through life trying to save.
Will Rogers, 1879–1935, Humorist and Showman

Chapter

19

Rest, Relaxation, and Rejuvenation

In this chapter we will explore the importance of rest, relaxation, and rejuvenation and some strategies for taking control. By the end of this chapter you will have created a plan for ensuring that you get needed rest, relaxation, and rejuvenation.

Rest

Do you get enough rest? Do you get regular vacations, or at least get a chance to change your routine? Why does it matter? Rest and relaxation is a far more important factor in our health than most of us realize.

Lack of sleep puts the body under stress and makes you vulnerable to a host of stress-related illnesses, such as colds and flu. It can even put you at risk for more serious illnesses, such as heart disease. You are especially vulnerable to illness during holidays or unusually stressful events because stress and lack of sleep go hand in hand. Did you know that getting by on just five hours or less of sleep two nights per week triples your risk of heart attack and doubles your risk for heart disease? Do you get enough sleep?

Why does lack of sleep make us vulnerable? Medical researchers believe that since sleep promotes healing, inadequate rest keeps the body from healing properly. With increasing evidence that inflammation and infection are major factors in heart disease, getting insufficient sleep puts you at increased risk. Insufficient sleep is not an unusual problem—nearly 70% of Americans surveyed by the National Sleep Foundation (http://www.sleepfoundation.org/) said that they experience frequent sleep problems. Sleep deprivation and sleep disorders were estimated to cost Americans $100 billion annually in medical expenses, sick leave, and lost productivity.

You may remember from Chapter 8 that sleeplessness is now being recognized as a symptom of heart disease. Participants in the National Institute of Health (NIH) study of women heart attack survivors recalled unusual fatigue (71%) and sleeplessness (48%) in the 30 days before their heart attacks. Is sleeplessness a symptom, or could not sleeping have kept their bodies from healing and brought on the heart attacks? We don't yet know. Sleeplessness could be a side effect from menopause or may be related to diet and exercise, but if you're dealing with sleeplessness, see your doctor right away. Don't put yourself at risk.

What about if you get enough hours of sleep, but it isn't restful? Those with sleep apnea, a condition that causes breathing to stop during sleep and leads to restless sleep, would seem to be at risk. That is indeed the case as sleep apnea has been associated with high blood pressure, heart disease, heart attack, and stroke.

How do you know if you have sleep apnea? One reason to suspect it might be if family members complain about your snoring. Another is if you get enough hours of sleep but don't feel rested. Or if you have difficulty sleeping. If so, talk to your doctor. He or she may suggest monitoring to determine if you actually have sleep apnea, either with a portable monitor that you wear to sleep or through monitoring at a sleep clinic. Approximately 18 million Americans suffer from sleep apnea, according to the National Institutes of Health. Solutions include weight loss or a breathing apparatus, called a C-PAP, which provides oxygen to promote restful sleep.

If you travel in your work, especially changing time zones frequently, sleep can be a big problem. After attending meetings all day, I usually took the late flight to the next location. Between arriving late, time zone changes, and the pace and stress of travel keeping me keyed up, it was hard to settle in and get to sleep, especially the first night. Some hotel beds were so uncomfortable that I simply couldn't sleep in them—the floor might have been more comfortable. I now carry a relaxation CD (see resources in Appendix B) in my computer to play when I want to nap while traveling and to sleep more restfully at my destination. And since most hotel beds are so lousy, I swear by Westin's Heavenly Bed—with its thick mattress, foam topper, and plush comforter and pillows, it is heavenly!

When I started traveling frequently to San Jose, I'd usually stay at the Westin in nearby Santa Clara. San Jose was sometimes moldy, and I'm very sensitive to molds. At home we run an air cleaner to clean the air of molds and provide "white noise." Since we live out in the country where it's quiet, the noisiness of hotels at night drives me crazy—as soon as you drop off to sleep, someone slams a door or yells and you're jarred awake. On one trip, I asked the front desk supervisor, Martina, if she could get an air cleaner for my room—for the cost of one night's stay she would have a loyal customer. When I returned that night, there was a HEPA air cleaner running in my room. From then on, when I checked into the hotel, my air cleaner was waiting for me. It removed molds from the air and provided white noise, significantly improving my sleep. It was a good investment for the hotel, and they got their money back because I stayed there about 200 nights over the next several years.

Getting enough sleep not only decreases your risk of heart attacks, but has also been proven to help you work more effectively and deal with difficult situations. A recent study in Germany (http://www.nature.com/nsu/040119/040119-10.html) found that those who got enough sleep—eight hours per night—could better solve problems.

Here are some simple strategies to maximize your rest, especially during stressful times such as the holidays when we're all so frazzled.

1) **Prioritize** what's most important to you and your family. Do what's most important, skip the rest, and don't feel guilty.

2) **Share the load** by recruiting family members to pitch in around the house.

3) **Give** to others in ways that boost your own spirits as well.

4) **Nap**, if possible, if you're feeling tired or run down, even if only for 10 minutes.

5) **Eat a healthy, balanced diet**, with lots of fruits and veggies, and avoid calorie-laden fast-foods.

6) **Drink water** throughout the day, but minimize during the last few hours before bedtime.

7) **Minimize caffeine**, and avoid it during the late afternoon and evening.

8) **Avoid sweets** just before bedtime to eliminate a sugar high.

9) **Exercise** during the day to ensure your body is tired at bedtime. You'll fall asleep faster and sleep longer.

10) **Create bedtime routines**—stick to a consistent bedtime, taking into account your body's rhythms. Have a bedtime ritual (brush teeth, remove makeup, apply night creams). Gently unwind by reading or listening to music for 30 minutes before going to bed, bringing the lights down gradually as you do so. I fall asleep to a relaxing CD.

11) **Check your bedding** to be sure you have a comfortable mattress and pillows, and the right covers to neither get too hot nor too cold.

You don't have to do all of the above—just pick a few to focus on, and don't stress over them.

Relaxation and Rejuvenation

It's not just rest or sleep that's important for your health. It's also relaxation and rejuvenation. Vacations are a good starting point. The Harvard Heart Letter in March, 2004, reported that two large studies indicate that those who get away live longer and are at less risk for heart disease.

Since I'm grounded and can't fly for now, we travel in our motorhome. It is relaxing and restful, and usually takes several weeks. Traveling in a motor home allows the mind to wander (while you're a passenger) and to think. Life is relaxed, and you see the country from a perch high above the traffic. I could live that way full time!

When I return, I'm more focused and productive. Work seems effortless. I come back full of ideas and the energy with which to execute them.

What about you? Do you regularly take time off to reset your perspective? Do you think you can't afford the time? Think again—can you afford not to?

Unlike the Europeans, Americans tend not to use up our vacation. Some of us just can't find time to take off; others fear what will happen when they return, such as whether there will be a job to come back to. Sure, there have been times where someone returned from work to find that his or her job had been eliminated. Many of us know someone to whom that has happened. Perhaps even you. But those cases are few and far between. I personally would be much more concerned that not getting away from work to reset and revitalize could lead to diminished effectiveness. Have you known someone for whom that was the case? Possibly more than one.

Not taking all of our vacation time may be a major factor in our high level of heart attacks. We need the time to let down and regroup, gaining a fresh perspective on life. I strongly encourage you to schedule vacation and to stick to it.

Take the time. You don't have to go someplace expensive or special—just get away from your routine, and especially from your stressors. Be careful not to overdo the pace on vacation though, causing you additional stress.

One stressor for many of us is the mountains of e-mail we receive while gone. Should you check it while you're gone? That's a matter of personal preference. You may prefer to pull e-mail while on vacation, so you don't stress out about dealing with an avalanche on your return; or you may prefer to stay away from it, and just deal with the onslaught later. I used to be in the first camp, but now tend toward the latter; plowing through it when I return seems less stressful than spending vacation time on it.

If you haven't gotten away recently from work, and e-mail, it's time to start planning for it. You need the time to focus on what's truly important to you, think about your future, and plan where you want to be. When you come up with the answers to those questions, write them down and focus on them. That resets your perspective, and puts you on the road to making them happen! You might be surprised at how much easier things are once you have that fresh perspective!

Take time, also, to see and live life fully. As I mentioned, on a flight right after my close call, I witnessed a glorious sunset over the Grand Canyon and set a goal to see it up close. We finally visited the Grand Canyon, and it was indeed spectacular.

Take the time to enjoy vacation—it's not a race. On the Grand Canyon trip, we also visited the Hoover Dam. While we were waiting in line for the dam tour, a father and young son behind us were looking at their map. We overheard the dad say, loudly, "Today, Las Vegas; tomorrow, Denver; next day, Chicago." As I wondered why someone would fly from city to city with the family and only spend a day in each, the son said, "Daddy, why do we have to drive. Why can't we fly?"

My jaw dropped—I was stunned. That's 1,700 miles, in just two days! That's a family vacation? Four hundred miles per day is plenty in my book. Instantly, my mind flashed to Chevy Chase in the movie, Vacation, as the Griswold family drove cross-country in their station wagon, hell-bent for WallyWorld. This was probably an off-the-scale driver carrying over work habits to vacation. What message was this kamikaze Dad giving his kid by overprogramming the family vacation? That's not restful.

Not long ago, I surveyed the subscribers to my Healthy Living News e-zine regarding their philosophies about vacations. I wanted to find out how important vacations were to them. I asked them to click on a link to send me an e-mail with the answer that most closely described their feelings about vacations.

Answers flooded in right away, and I was surprised that about one-third said they always took vacations, another third tried to but weren't always able to, and the remaining third said that they couldn't find the time. However, when many of the subscribers returned from their own vacations and replied, the distribution shifted significantly. The final results are in Figure 19.1 below.

Vacation Survey Results	
Choice	Response
I always take regular vacations as they're important to me	65%
I try to take regular vacations, but sometimes must reschedule	20%
I cannot find time for vacation	15%

Figure 19.1: Vacation Survey Results

I also asked for comments, and it was great to hear how important vacation is for most. Some of them take regular cruises, so they can't be tracked down by cell phone or e-mail. Some go to places they've never seen, such as Kenya, South Africa, China, Denmark, England, and France. One goes someplace new for every birthday. Another spends three weeks in Europe each year, and has for 20 years. Others take frequent short breaks, still getting away from the routine. Many go to see family, entertain family, or get away together as a family at places such as the beach. I thought you might find their comments interesting, so I've included them in Figure 19.2

Vacation Comments

When I surveyed subscribers to my e-zine, they shared a lot of wisdom about vacations.

I practically mandate that at least one vacation per year is done via a cruise. It gives me a great excuse to be totally disconnected since Internet access charges and cell phone capabilities are very costly when you're traveling by cruise ship. I also like the stress-reducing aspects of having my food and lodging stay dependable and consistent while I visit multiple places (often multiple countries). It's really nice to unpack just once for the whole time, even though I'm going to multiple locations.

I'm such a fan of cruising that I could probably become a cruise consultant as a second career path. Last summer we took a Baltic cruise that stopped in Norway, Sweden, Finland, Russia, Estonia, and Denmark. Talk about a fantastic voyage! This summer we're taking a second cruise to Alaska. Since the ship departs right from Seattle, we don't even have to do any flying at either end of the cruise. Way cool!

--Karlene Seime-Noble, Financial industry executive

Every summer I have my niece and nephew down for a week. Although it's not "relaxing" per se, it is a definite diversion from work. We swim, we bike ride, and we go places and do lots of interesting things. I usually go back to work totally worn out. However, it does provide a different kind of exhaustion from the mental stress of work. I do not answer email or give work a thought during this week.

--Brandy Meeks, Texas state government agency

Since I turned 50 last year, I have vowed to take a minimum of two weeks off at a time and to NOT check my emails until I get back!

Vacation Comments

Furthermore, I vowed that every year on the date of my birth, I will be in a place I have never seen before. This year it will be a trip to our country's capitol—Washington DC.

--Carla Daws, Texas state government agency

I was raised in a family that traveled throughout the United States. I have been to 49 (Wisconsin is missing) of the 50 states. It gave me a lifetime passion for traveling. I have taken a vacation away from my home state every year of my life and I am currently 55.

For the past twenty years, I have spent three consecutive weeks a year in Europe. Although I had a stressful job, I knew that those three weeks were MINE. A vacation always recharged my batteries and I was much more effective when I returned. Work, phone, and emails can be delegated and/or WAIT.

Although I have been in an extended job search, my vacation planning and vacations continue.

--Jeanie Meyer

We take family vacations, even with our grown kids and elderly parents. It's a great opportunity for quality time together.

Our favorite place is the beach. For many years, we have rented a condo for a week at South Padre. We like a big home-cooked breakfast, and then the rest of the day is totally unstructured. Some choose to swim, walk the beach, sleep, read, etc, etc, ...just whatever makes your day.

It's been challenging at times to synchronize schedules with kids in college, work schedules, etc., but everyone obviously values the time enough to make it a priority.

--Jo Rake, Healthcare industry executive

When I was working, vacations were something I never had time for. When I actually was let go from my job, I had almost 4 weeks of vacation! The vacation I had back then was used for my children's sick time; as a single parent that was it for vacation. I guess the irony of life is I worked all those years to raise my children anticipating time for myself for those vacations and to complete my educational goal!

Now that I am unemployed, it will be a long while before I have a vacation. I would be lying if I said this does not bother me. I really was looking forward to this time in my life.

--Tammy, Austin, TX

I just cannot find time for vacation. Actually, my reason is that being single, I do not want to go alone.
A couple of weeks later: I just wanted to say hi and thank you again for always sending your newsletters. Great reminders that I need to change my diet at times. I am actually typing from the plane—just spent four days in Kauai. I am trying to take your advice :) Good news is I did take time off from work.

--Anonymous high-tech employee

Figure 19.2: Vacation Comments

What about you? What type of vacation do you like? A spa, beach, or mountain vacation? An intellectual or academic vacation? *Please share your own vacation thoughts and experiences with me—send them to info@saveherlife.com, and please put the book title in your subject line so that your message doesn't inadvertently land in the spam filter.*

It generally takes time to get a big vacation on the schedule and to get away. In the meantime, you can take mini-vacations, and perhaps make some changes that can make you more effective.

Another source of rejuvenation is having outside interests—volunteering, social support among friends, church responsibilities and interests, and hobbies. By providing balance and relieving stress, these outside interests and social connections increase optimism and health. Research has confirmed that those with social support have lower health risks.

Please take care of yourself. If you're out of balance, or are a Type A, like me, please take back control so that you get enough rest and exercise. Take seriously the need to take time to play and de-stress. Allow yourself the time to think and reflect—it's not a luxury, it's a necessity. Work-life balance is hard to achieve, but is so vitally important to your health. There are a lot of people counting on you. Please take care of you.

> *When I think of talking, it is of course with a woman. For talking at its best being an inspiration, it wants a corresponding divine quality of receptiveness, and where will you find this but in a woman?*
> Oliver Wendell Holmes, 1809–1894, Author and Physician

Create Your Rest, Relaxation, and Rejuvenation Plan

It's time to create your plan for rest, relaxation, and rejuvenation. Start by answering these questions, in Figure 19.3, to create your goals.

1) How much sleep do I need?

2) What are my risks from not getting enough sleep?

3) How can I ensure that I get enough sleep?

4) What are some of the ways I plan to relax?

5) What are my philosophies regarding vacations, including what I like to do and where I like to go for vacation?

6) What are my plans for vacation or getting away?

7) How will I commit to do these things?

8) What benefits will I see from doing them?

9) What will I do to rejuvenate my mind, spirit, and body?

Rest, Relaxation, and Rejuvenation Goals
How much sleep do I need?
What are my risks from not getting enough sleep?
How can I ensure that I get enough sleep?
What are some of the ways I plan to relax?
What are my philosophies regarding vacations, including what I like to do and where I like to go for vacation?
What are my plans for vacation or getting away?
How will I commit to do these things?
What benefits will I see from doing them?
What will I do to rejuvenate my mind, spirit, and body?

Figure 19.3: Your Rest, Relaxation, and Rejuvenation Goals

In Figure 19.4 is a sample Rest, Relaxation, and Rejuvenation Plan based on goals defined in a sample version of Figure 19.3 (not shown). For each area to be addressed, the current situation and ideal situation are listed along with steps to get from current to ideal and target dates to do so.

Rest, Relaxation, and Rejuvenation Plan and Targets

Area to Address	Current	Ideal	Commitments/ Action Steps	Target Dates
Rest	5–6 hrs/night	7–8 hrs/night	Increase sleep	2 weeks
Relaxation	Infrequent vacations	Vacation/ quarter	Schedule vacation	3 months
Rejuvenation		Spa vacation each yr	Spa for long weekend	6 months
Rejuvenation	Infrequent massages	Bi-weekly massage	Schedule massage	2 weeks

Figure 19.4: Sample Rest, Relaxation, and Rejuvenation Plan

Using your goals in Figure 19.3, create your own Rest, Relaxation, and Rejuvenation Plan in Figure 19.5, below. Identify areas to address, your current and ideal states, and your commitment and target dates.

Rest, Relaxation, and Rejuvenation Plan and Targets

Area to Address	Current	Ideal	Commitments/ Action Steps	Target Dates

Figure 19.5: Your Rest, Relaxation, and Rejuvenation Plan and Targets

Now that you have created your plan for rest, relaxation, and rejuvenation, let's look at how to take proactive control of your health, in Chapter 20.

An unhurried sense of time is in itself a form of wealth.
Bonnie Friedman, Author

Chapter

20

Take Proactive Control of Your Health

In this chapter we'll explore ways to educate yourself about your health, how to partner with your health care provider, and what kind of regular checkups to get. By the end of this chapter you will have created a plan for taking proactive control of your health.

You are responsible for your own health. No one else is. If you don't take care of yourself, who will?

In previous chapters, you identified life changes necessary for optimum health. How, then, can you best ensure that good health? Don't rely on luck for it—most of us won't be as lucky as one 67-year old grandmother was recently. In traveling from her home in Britain to her daughter's wedding in Florida, she was on a flight to Orlando when she experienced back, chest, and arm pains, sweating, and vomiting, and realized that she was having a heart attack. When the flight attendant called to see if there was a doctor on board, fifteen cardiologists answered the call. All were headed to a cardiology conference in Orlando. They were able to save her, and the plane landed in North Carolina, where she spent 5 days in the hospital before proceeding to Orlando for her daughter's wedding.

She was lucky, but luck doesn't cut it for most of us. Here are some specific steps we can take to optimize our health: educating ourselves about our health, partnering with our healthcare providers, and getting regular checkups. We'll talk about each of these, starting with educating ourselves.

Educate Yourself

With the resources available to us today, especially on the Internet, it's much easier than ever to know what is happening in the medical and healthcare fields, and I encourage you to do so. However, it's easy to get overwhelmed. And what about quality? Some information on the Internet is just plain wrong, and other information is suspect. There are, however, many trustworthy Internet health and medical resources, some of which I've listed in Figure 20.1. These are all great resources.

Internet Health and Medical Resources

❑ American Heart Association
http://www.americanheart.org

❑ American Heart Association Journals—*Circulation*, *Hypertension*, and *Stroke*
http://www.ahajournals.org/

Internet Health and Medical Resources

- American Stroke Association
  http://www.strokeassociation.org

- Berkeley Wellness Letter
  http://www.berkeleywellness.com/

- Cleveland Clinic Heart Center
  http://www.clevelandclinic.org/heartcenter/

- CNN Health
  http://www.cnn.com/HEALTH/

- Harvard Medical School Health Letters
  http://www.health.harvard.edu/hhp/index.jsp

- Heart Center Online for Patients
  http://www.heartcenteronline.com/myheartdr/home/index.cfm

- Johns Hopkins Medicine
  http://www.hopkinsmedicine.org/HealthInformation/index.html

- Karolinska Institute Library—Diseases, Disorders, and Related Topics
  http://www.mic.ki.se/Diseases/index.html

- Mayo Clinic Consumer Health
  http://www.mayoclinic.com/index.cfm

- Medem—Sponsored by 45 medical societies, including the American Medical Association
  http://www.medem.com/index.cfm

- MEDLINEplus
  U.S. National Library of Medicine and the National Institutes of Health
  http://medlineplus.gov/

- Medscape and WebMD
  http://www.webmd.com/

- MedWebPlus—Global health science index by topic and region
  http://www.medwebplus.com/

- National Health Service (UK)
  http://www.nhs.uk/

- Nature—Medical and scientific topics
  http://www.nature.com/

- University of California Berkeley Library's Public Health Resources
  http://www.lib.berkeley.edu/PUBL/internet.html

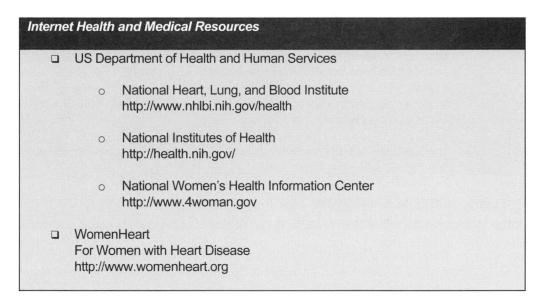

Figure 20.1: Internet Health and Medical Resources

While I encourage you to be proactive by doing your homework and staying on top of what is happening in medical research, I know that in reality you probably don't have the time to do this regularly. Most of us already have way too much to do. That's where I can help. I comb the medical research and publish a bi-weekly Healthy Living News e-zine (e-mail newsletter) that shares the latest in medical research and health tips. If you'd like to receive this resource, simply sign up by clicking on the **Newsletter** button at **http://www.SaveHerLife.com**. When you get the e-zine, please pass it along to others that can benefit.

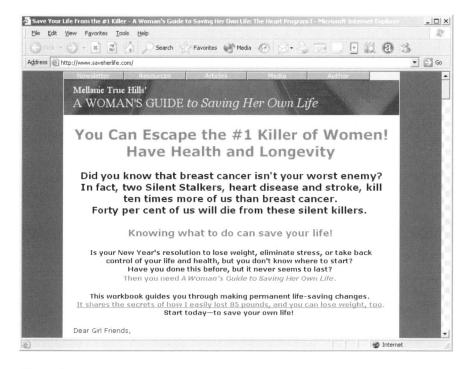

Figure 20.2: Resources Available at http://www.SaveHerLife.com

You'll also find the resources listed in Appendix B of this book by clicking on the **Resources** button at **http://www.SaveHerLife.com**. By clicking on the **Articles** button at **http://www.SaveHerLife.com** you'll find the health articles I've written or articles for which I've been interviewed as well as the archives of my Healthy Living News e-zine. Previous issues of the e-zine focused on medical research updates, cholesterol, diets, exercise, stress, anger, sleep, vacations, heart health, aging, hormone replacement therapy (HRT), and breast cancer.

The next step in taking proactive control of your health is partnering with your healthcare provider.

Partner With Your Health Care Provider

Doctors are so busy today that we can't expect them to guess when something is wrong with us. We have to pay attention to our own symptoms, and do something about them, working with our doctors to figure it all out.

I would expect that the majority of doctors believe that the best patients are those who are informed and ask the right questions. If you have done your homework, and can go in to see your doctor with a focused list of questions, you're more likely to have a good outcome. If your doctor doesn't like you asking lots of questions, then maybe you're not seeing the right doctor.

Write down your questions beforehand so that you don't forget to ask something at your appointment. Keep a running list of topics and questions, and take that with you. At your next visit, take your risk assessments from Figures 7.9 and 15.2 to discuss with your doctor. Talk about your risk factors and decide together what further tests, if any, to do. Identify any other areas of concern upon which to focus.

Your doctor may not specifically discuss heart disease with you, especially if you're young. Why do I say that? Because one study found that just 14 percent of women ages 25 to 34 had heard from their doctors about heart disease, and among women aged 35 to 44, only 27 per cent. Be proactive and ask about it.

There was a recent newspaper article indicating that ob-gyns often don't discuss with their patients a new procedure for treating fibroids, and instead focus on more expensive and invasive hysterectomies. The article hinted at conspiracy by ob-gyns. There may be some doctors that fall into that camp, but most want to do what's best for their patients. They may be struggling with information overload and are squeezed by a health care system that is totally out of control. Therefore, it's in our best interest to be informed and knowledgeable patients.

Let's talk next about getting regular checkups.

Get Regular Check-ups

We need to make sure to get regular checkups, especially as we reach menopause. Do you have a family physician or general practitioner, or do you only see an ob-gyn? Many ob-gyns treat the whole person, but that is not the case with all of them. If your ob-gyn is only focused on the bikini areas (breasts and reproductive systems), and doesn't probe about other areas such as your heart, you may not be getting the whole-body focus that you need. Consider seeing a family physician or general practitioner as well. Your doctors should be working together, so as I refer to your "doctor" below, think in terms of your health care team.

What should you expect in doctor visits? According to many doctors, if you're not getting your blood pressure and weight checked, and your doctor doesn't ask about your family history and check for other risk factors, then you're not receiving proper care.

From this book, you've learned the symptoms and risk factors for heart disease and stroke, so discuss any symptoms or concerns with your doctor. Your doctor will probably order cholesterol tests, not just for total cholesterol, but also for HDL, LDL, and triglycerides. Cholesterol tests are easy—just a simple blood test requiring a few hours of fasting.

Your doctor may also order other blood tests if you have multiple risk factors or have symptoms. Newer tests, such as homocysteine and C-Reactive Protein, hold great promise for identifying heart disease risk, but are not yet widely in use.

If you have strong symptoms, your doctor can administer a simple and quick EKG (electrocardiogram) or send you for a stress test. If a stress test indicates a problem, the next step is a heart scan or cardiac catheterization, as we discussed in Chapter 9. For a catheterization, the doctor places a tiny slit in the artery in your upper leg, inserts a catheter into the artery, and pumps in dye to watch the blood flow via a special screen. (Don't worry, you're under anesthesia and won't feel it.) This is how we found my blockage.

One doctor told me that most women should be taking a low-dose baby aspirin (81 mg) each day to make the blood platelets less sticky so they don't clot and cause a heart attack. Ask your doctor if you should do that. Some people may be at risk and shouldn't take aspirin, and others don't respond to aspirin. Aspirin non-responsiveness is thought to be caused by smoking, overweight, high cholesterol, and high blood pressure.

It's not just about your heart though. There are other tests to consider, too, such as a breast self-exam, Pap smear, mammogram, bone density scan, flexible sigmoidoscopy (or maybe a colonoscopy), and lots more. Some may be done by your ob-gyn, and others by your family physician. Ask your doctors what tests you should be getting, and how often. That can vary depending on family history. If you have had one, or more, female relative(s) with breast cancer, you will need to be on a more frequent and aggressive program of testing and tracking, and may even want to consider genetic testing for you and other family members.

If you don't get answers and solutions from your doctor, seek a second opinion. Some doctors were trained when heart disease wasn't a woman's issue, so they don't know what to look for in women and may mistake your symptoms as simply being something else. What your doctor doesn't know can hurt you, so it's important to be a proactive member of your own health care team.

A couple of issues unique to women are hormone replacement therapy and mammograms, so I've included some facts in Figure 20.3 about hormone replacement therapy (HRT) and in Figure 20.4 about mammograms.

Hormone Replacement Therapy

Whether or not to use hormone replacement therapy (HRT) is an important concern for any woman approaching, in, and beyond, menopause. The findings revealed recently raise increased doubts about the use of HRT for anything other than short-term relief of menopausal symptoms.

Until recently, doctors prescribed HRT not only for the relief of menopausal symptoms, such as hot flashes, but also for HRT's protective effect against heart disease, colon cancer, and osteoporosis. If your family history included those conditions, HRT was advised to provide protection against them, though the downside was an increase in the risk of breast cancer.

That all changed in mid-2002 when data from the Women's Health Initiative (WHI), a study sponsored by the National Institutes of Health, indicated that women using Prempro™—a type of HRT combining estrogen and progestin—were at increased risk of heart disease, stroke, and blood clots. As a result, many women discontinued their use of HRT.

Women on estrogen-only HRT—those who have had hysterectomies—were counseled to bide their time since the second part of the WHI study, on estrogen-only Premarin®, was continuing. Now, however, that study has just been stopped, a year early, further challenging our beliefs about HRT. The essential question being pursued, whether estrogen-only HRT protects the heart, had been answered—the expected protective effect was not seen. Estrogen-only HRT neither increased, nor decreased, study participant's risk of heart disease, but did result in a slight increase in stroke risk. For that reason, researchers discontinued the study, moving into the follow-up stages. Quite surprisingly, no increase in breast cancer risk was seen in this study. Both studies showed a reduced risk of hip fractures, so HRT is valuable for those at greatest risk of osteoporosis.

Since estrogen-plus-progestin HRT increased heart disease risk, and estrogen-only HRT showed no difference, one likely conjecture is that estrogen's impact on our hearts is neutral, and progestin's impact is negative, but that calls into question the long-held belief that women have been less vulnerable prior to menopause because our bodies make estrogens. Or perhaps the difference is between the estrogens our bodies make and those from outside the body.

So what does that mean to us? If you use HRT, you should discuss these findings with your doctor and identify the potential HRT risks/benefits for you. Since many of the women in the study were in their sixties when the study began, the meaning for younger women is still unknown.

Of course, at issue now is what we should do about menopause symptoms. The FDA recommends using estrogens and progestins in the lowest possible amounts, and for the shortest possible time, so they still advise it for short-term use. For some of us, though, that isn't an option, so we suffer through hot flashes and sleeplessness when we go off HRT, or until we find other forms of hormones that work for us. That leads us to wonder whether the sleeplessness we experience is from going off HRT or is related to sleeplessness as a symptom of heart disease. That's yet another reason that it's hard for women to know if they are experiencing symptoms from heart disease or from something else.

When the study started, hormone options were more limited, but there are now many non-oral forms available. Do the study's results apply just to the oral forms of hormone

Hormone Replacement Therapy

replacement therapy? We don't have those answers, but they're certainly worth investigating.

Recently, scientists in Scandinavia called off their HRT study among women who had already experienced breast cancer due to the high risk of breast cancer recurrence among study participants.

Deciding whether or not to be on hormone replacement therapy is something with which women and their doctors will continue to struggle.

Figure 20.3: Hormone Replacement Therapy

Mammograms

Should you have regular mammograms, and how frequently? Here are some facts that can help in making that decision.

❑ For women over age fifty, having a mammogram annually saves lives due to a 30% reduction in death rates from breast cancer. Women in their forties showed a 16%–18% reduction in mortality rates.

❑ The American Cancer Society and the National Cancer Institute recommend starting to have mammograms at age 40, and to have them every one–two years.

❑ Mammograms aren't as accurate for pre-menopausal women because their breast tissue is denser, resulting in a higher rate of false positives. For example, 97% of women in their forties who underwent surgical biopsies resulting from the findings on their mammograms didn't actually have breast cancer.

❑ Specific factors that put you at risk for breast cancer include having a close relative who has had breast cancer, having your first child in your thirties or later, not having children, early menstrual cycles (before age twelve), and being African American. Diet can also put you at risk, as can antibiotic use.

❑ According to a new study, antibiotic users had a 50% higher risk of breast cancer, and the higher the use, the higher the risk. Researchers believed that the antibiotic use was linked to chronic inflammation, which was linked to cancer and heart disease.

Figure 20.4: Mammograms

Create Your Plan for Taking Proactive Control of Your Health

In order to create a plan to take proactive control of your health, answer these questions in Figure 20.5.

1) What will I commit to doing to stay updated on the latest in medical research and health care? How will I do these things? What benefits will I see from doing them?

2) What can I do to better partner with my healthcare providers?

3) How often do I need to get checkups? When will I get my next checkup? What are my health concerns, and what do I need to discuss with my healthcare provider?

Plan for Taking Proactive Control of My Health

1. Educate Myself
    What will I commit to doing to stay updated on the latest in medical research and health care? How will I do these things? What benefits will I see from doing them?

2. Partner With My Healthcare Providers
    What can I do to better partner with my healthcare providers?

3. Get Regular Check-ups
    How often do I need to get checkups? When will I get my next checkup? What are my health concerns, and what do I need to discuss with my healthcare provider?

Figure 20.5: Your Plan for Taking Proactive Control of Your Health

Now that we have created a set of plans for our health using the HEART Program, let's put this all together, in Chapter 21.

Putting It All Together and Making a Commitment

Now that you have completed your plan, you're at least halfway there. Putting it down on paper makes it so much more tangible and real, and puts you well on your way to optimum health and longevity. I hope that you're now ready to start acting on your plan.

The next step is to put the goals in your plan on your calendar so that you can hold yourself accountable. You might consider having an ***accountability partner***, someone supportive who will help you and encourage you to meet your goals. Even better would be for your accountability partner to be working through her own HEART plan, too. That way, you can hold each other mutually accountable. This book would make a great gift for the other special women in your life.

I've been your partner throughout the process, and would like to continue to be your partner. Since it takes twenty-one days to create a new habit, and by the thirtieth day it should be established as a permanent part of your life, please e-mail me on day thirty at HEART@saveherlife.com to let me know how it's going (please add that to your goal calendar). Please share your results and send me your feedback or testimonials about the book, process, and tools. I'd appreciate your input on ways to improve it, and let me know of any topics or questions to address in my Healthy Living News e-zine or in subsequent books. I want to help you on your journey to a lifetime of good health.

As a coach, I'll be glad to provide additional help through this process. Just send me an e-mail or give me a call. I'm offering readers of this book a special 20% discount on coaching.

As you move forward in implementing your plan, remember the words of Robert Frost in his poem, The Road Not Taken. In it, he spoke of how taking the road less traveled had made all the difference. You have a choice—choose health. Take the road to responsibility for your life and your health—that can make all the difference. Create the life you wish to lead.

I wish you the best. Have a long, happy, healthy life.

Mellanie True Hills
512-267-5610
HEART@saveherlife.com
http://www.SaveHerLife.com

Appendix A: Master Forms

Risk Assessment				
Risk Factor/Measures	Current	Normal / Ideal	Risk Y/N	Risk Count
Age _____				
Gender _____				
1. Smoking	_____	No_____	____	____
2. Diabetes	_____		____	____
Blood glucose	_____	7%, or less_____		
3. Blood pressure	_____	120/80, or less____	____	____
4. Cholesterol	_____		____	____
Total		Under 200_____		
Triglycerides		Under 150_____		
LDL (Bad)	_____	Under 130, or under 70 in heart patients		
HDL (Good)	_____	Over 50_____		
5. Family history	_____	No_____	____	____
6. Overweight	_____		____	____
Height	_____			
Weight	_____	See Figure 7.5_____		
BMI	_____	Less than 25_____		
Waist circumference	_____	Less than 35 inches_		
Weight classification	_____	Normal_____		
Risk (BMI & waist)	_____	See Figure 7.6_____		
7. Activity level	_____	Moderate to active__	____	____
8. Stress	_____	Controlled/managed_	____	____
9. Other risks/measures			____	____
_____	_____	_____		
_____	_____	_____		
_____	_____	_____		
Total Risks				____

Figure 7.9: Your Risk Assessment

Question 1: What Are My Values?

1. _____
2. _____
3. _____
4. _____
5. _____
6. _____
7. _____
8. _____
9. _____
10. _____
11. _____
12. _____

Figure 14.2: Your Answers To Question 1, What Are My Values?

Question 2: What Are My Ideal and Actual Priorities?

Ideal	Actual
1. _____	1. _____
2. _____	2. _____
3. _____	3. _____
4. _____	4. _____
5. _____	5. _____
6. _____	6. _____
7. _____	7. _____

Figure 14.4: Your Answers to Question 2, What Are My Ideal and Actual Priorities?

Question 3: What Would My Ideal Life Look Like?

1. _____
2. _____
3. _____
4. _____
5. _____
6. _____
7. _____

Figure 14.6: Your Answers to Question 3, What Would My Ideal Life Look Like?

Question 4: How Do I Attain My Ideal Life?

Actual

Ideal

How to Bridge the Gap

Figure 14.8: Your Answers to Question 4, How Do I Attain My Ideal Life?

Question 5: When Can I Attain My Ideal Life?

Goals / Objectives

Completion Date

Figure 14.10: Your Answers to Question 5, When Can I Attain My Ideal Life?

HEART Program Action Plan						
Risk Factor/ Measures	Risk	Current	Ideal/ Goal	Gap	Action/ Step(s)	Target Date
1. Smoking	—					
2. Diabetes Blood glucose	—					
3. Blood pressure	—					
4. Cholesterol Total Triglycerides LDL (Bad) HDL (Good)	—					
5. Family history	—					
6. Overweight Height Weight (1st goal) BMI Waist Weight class Risk (BMI/waist) Weight (2nd goal)	—					
7. Activity level	—					
8. Stress	—					
9. Other	—					

Figure 15.2: Your HEART Program Action Plan

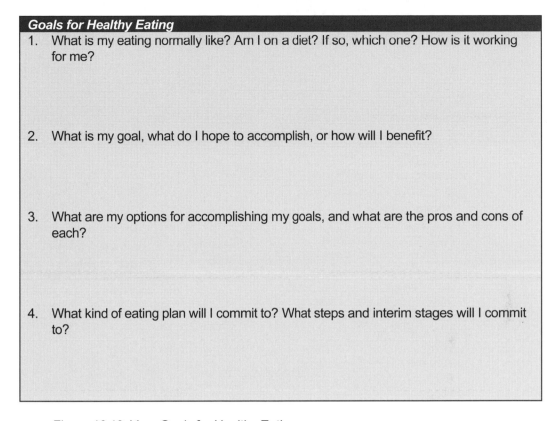

Goals for Healthy Eating

1. What is my eating normally like? Am I on a diet? If so, which one? How is it working for me?

2. What is my goal, what do I hope to accomplish, or how will I benefit?

3. What are my options for accomplishing my goals, and what are the pros and cons of each?

4. What kind of eating plan will I commit to? What steps and interim stages will I commit to?

Figure 16.10: Your Goals for Healthy Eating

Healthy Eating Plan and Targets				
Food Groups	Current Servings Per Day	Ideal Servings Per Day	Commitments/ Action Steps	Target Dates
Breads, cereals, and pasta		5–6 (1-oz)		
Fruits		3 (½ c)		
Vegetables, made up of: Dark-green: 1½–3 c/wk Orange: 1–2 c/wk Legumes: 1–3 c/wk Starchy: 2½–3 c/wk Other: 4½–6½ c/wk		3–5 (½ c)		
Meat, poultry, fish, nuts, and seeds		4–5 oz		
Milk, yogurt, and cheese (fat-free)		2–3 cups		
Eggs		0–1 egg		
Fats and oils Oils: 18–22 g Solid fats: 12–14 g		30–36 g		
Discretionary calories		USDA 2005 Guidelines		

Figure 16.11: Your Healthy Eating Plan and Targets

Exercise Goals

1. What is my current exercise program like? How is it working for me?

2. What is my goal, what do I hope to accomplish, or how will I benefit?

3. What are my options for accomplishing my exercise goals, and what are the pros and cons of each?

4. What kind of exercise plan can I commit to? What will I do, and when will I do it? What is required (equipment, classes, gym membership, etc.) in order to accomplish it? What steps and interim stages will I commit to?

5. How will I know that I'm successful?

Figure 17.1: Your Exercise Goals

Exercise Plan and Targets

Exercise Program	Current	Ideal	Commitments/ Action Steps	Target Dates

Figure 17.3: Your Exercise Plan and Targets

Personal Stress Profile

What's my work stress level?

1 (Low)   (High) 10

What's my personal stress level?

1 (Low)   (High) 10

Figure 18.4: Your Personal Stress Profile

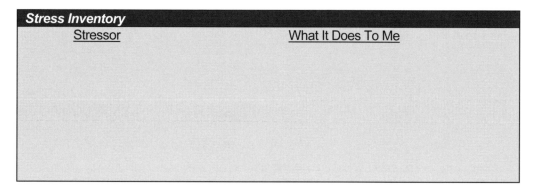

Stress Inventory

Stressor   What It Does To Me

Figure 18.6: Your Personal Stress Inventory

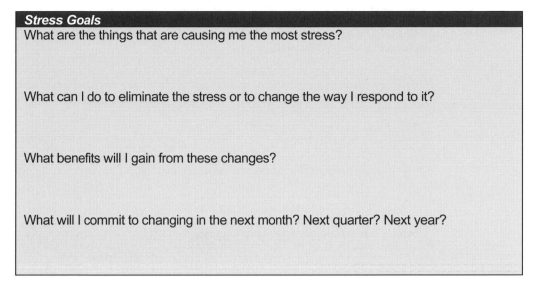

Stress Goals

What are the things that are causing me the most stress?

What can I do to eliminate the stress or to change the way I respond to it?

What benefits will I gain from these changes?

What will I commit to changing in the next month? Next quarter? Next year?

Figure 18.7: Your Personal Stress Goals

Stress Plan/Targets

Stressor	Current	Ideal	Commitments/ Action Steps	Target Dates

Figure 18.9: Your Stress Plan and Targets

Rest, Relaxation, and Rejuvenation Goals

How much sleep do I need?

What are my risks from not getting enough sleep?

How can I ensure that I get enough sleep?

What are some of the ways I plan to relax?

What are my philosophies regarding vacations, including what I like to do and where I like to go for vacation?

What are my plans for vacation or getting away?

How will I commit to do these things?

What benefits will I see from doing them?

What will I do to rejuvenate my mind, spirit, and body?

Figure 19.3: Your Rest, Relaxation, and Rejuvenation Goals

Rest, Relaxation, and Rejuvenation Plan and Targets				
Area to Address	Current	Ideal	Commitments/ Action Steps	Target Dates

Figure 19.5: Your Rest, Relaxation, and Rejuvenation Plan and Targets

Plan for Taking Proactive Control of My Health

1. Educate Myself
    What will I commit to doing to stay updated on the latest in medical research and health care? How will I do these things? What benefits will I see from doing them?

2. Partner With My Healthcare Providers
    What can I do to better partner with my healthcare providers?

3. Get Regular Check-ups
    How often do I need to get checkups? When will I get my next checkup? What are my health concerns, and what do I need to discuss with my healthcare provider?

Figure 20.5: Your Plan for Taking Proactive Control of Your Health

Appendix B: Resources

Resources Available at My Web Site

1) Many of the resources discussed in this book, including the items listed below and the Other Resources listed in the next section, can be found by clicking on **Resources** at **http://www.SaveHerLife.com**

   o *Achieve Your Chosen Weight*, *Relieve Stress*, *Restful Sleep*, *Relax and Succeed*, and *Overcome Anxiety* tape and CD programs

   o Brian Tracy resources

   o No Pudge Brownies

   o Joseph's Fat-Free Cookies

   o Healthy Travel Network's Travel Fit Kit and Hotel Room Workout

2) Health articles can be found by clicking on **Articles** at **http://www.SaveHerLife.com**

3) Past issues of my Healthy Living Newsletter (e-zine) as well as the link to subscribe to it can be found by selecting **Newsletter** at **http://www.SaveHerLife.com**

Other Resources Listed Throughout The Book

1) Activity Calorie Calculator
   http://www.primusweb.com/fitnesspartner/jumpsite/calculat.htm

2) American Association of Nutritional Sciences
   http://www.nutrition.org/

3) American Dietetic Association
   http://www.eatright.org/Public/

4) American Heart Association
   http://www.americanheart.org
   Food Pyramid
   http://www.deliciousdecisions.org/ee/afp.html
   Journals: Circulation, Hypertension, Stroke, and others
   http://www.ahajournals.org/

5) American Stroke Association
   http://www.strokeassociation.org

6) Berkeley Wellness Letter
http://www.berkeleywellness.com/

7) Cleveland Clinic
http://www.clevelandclinic.org/heartcenter/pub/guide/
Heart Center
http://www.clevelandclinic.org/heartcenter/

8) CNN Health
http://www.cnn.com/HEALTH/

9) Collage Designer Consignment Boutique
http://www.shopcollage.com

10) Dallas Dietetic Association Calorie Calculator
http://www.dallasdietitian.com/resources/calcalc.htm

11) European Society of Cardiology 2004
http://www.escardio.org/

12) Harvard Medical School Health Letters
http://www.health.harvard.edu/hhp/index.jsp

13) Heart Center Online for Patients
http://www.heartcenteronline.com/myheartdr/home/index.cfm

14) Institute of Medicine
Created by the US government
http://www.iom.edu/

15) Johns Hopkins Medicine
http://www.hopkinshospital.org/health_infol

16) Journal of the American College of Nutrition
http://www.jacn.org/

17) Journal of Experimental Psychology
http://www.apa.org/journals/xhp.html

18) Journal of Personality and Social Psychology
http://www.apa.org/journals/psp.html

19) Karolinska Institute Library
Diseases, disorders, and related topics
http://www.mic.ki.se/Diseases/index.html

20) Mayo Clinic Consumer Health
http://www.mayoclinic.com/
Food and Nutrition Center contains serving size guides, calorie counters, food
pyramids, and special diets
http://www.mayoclinic.com/findinformation/conditioncenters/centers.cfm?objectid
=000851DA-6222-1B37-8D7E80C8D77A0000

Mayo Clinic Proceedings
http://www.mayoclinic.com/invoke.cfm?id=MC00014

21) Medem
Sponsored by 45 medical societies, including the American Medical Association
http://www.medem.com/

22) Medline Plus
U.S. National Library of Medicine and National Institutes of Health
http://medlineplus.gov/

23) Medscape and WebMD
http://www.webmd.com/

24) MedWebPlus
Global health science index by topic and region
http://www.medwebplus.com/

25) National Association of Resale and Thrift Shops
http://www.narts.org/shopping/

26) National Health Service (UK)
http://www.nhs.uk/

27) National Heart, Lung, and Blood Institute
http://www.nhlbi.nih.gov/health
BMI Calculator at http://nhlbisupport.com/bmi
Classification of Overweight and Obesity at
http://www.nhlbi.nih.gov/health/public/heart/obesity/lose_wt/bmi_dis.htm

28) National Institutes of Health (US)
http://health.nih.gov/

29) National Sleep Foundation
http://www.sleepfoundation.org/

30) National Women's Health Information Center
http://www.4woman.gov

31) Nature
http://www.nature.com/

32) Parenting Your Parents
http://www.ParentingYourParents.com

33) Partnership for Essential Nutrition
http://www.essentialnutrition.org/

34) Sleep study in Germany
http://www.nature.com/nsu/040119/040119-10.html

35) Subway Nutrition Information
http://www.subway.com/applications/NutritionInfo/index.aspx

36) University of California Berkeley Library's
Public Health Resources on the Internet
http://www.lib.berkeley.edu/PUBL/internet.html

37) University of Illinois Champaign/Urbana Nutrition Analysis Tool
Analyze foods you eat, including fast foods
http://nat.crgq.com/index.html

38) US Department of Agriculture (USDA)

- Dietary Guidelines
  http://www.health.gov/dietaryguidelines/

- Food and Nutrition Information Center
  http://www.nal.usda.gov/fnic/etext/000108.html

- Interactive Healthy Eating Index
  Dietary assessment tool
  http://209.48.219.53/default.asp

- Nutrient Database Search
  http://www.nal.usda.gov/fnic/foodcomp/search/

- Nutritive Value of Foods
  Exhaustive list of foods and nutrient values
  http://www.nal.usda.gov/fnic/foodcomp/Data/HG72/hg72.html

39) WomenHeart
For women with heart disease
http://www.womenheart.org

Index

Quick Order Form

💻 Online: http://www.SaveHerLife.com. E-book and print books—order by credit card.

☎ Telephone orders: Call 877-432-7820 (877-HEART20) with your credit card.

🖨 Fax orders: Call 877-432-7820 to get number to fax this form.

✎ E-mail orders: orders@saveherlife.com

🖃 Postal orders: Mellanie True Hills, Healthy Ideas Press, P.O. Box 541, Greenwood, TX 76246 Telephone: 940-466-9898

❑ Please send _____ copies of A Woman's Guide to Saving Her Own Life. I understand that I may return them for a full refund – no questions asked.

❑ Please send FREE information on Speaking/Seminars.

Name_____

Address_____

City_____ State_____ Zip_____-____

Telephone_____

E-mail address_____

Sales tax: Please add 8.25% for products shipped to Texas addresses.

Shipping:
US $5 per book
International: $10 for first book; $6 for each additional book (estimate)

Payment: ❑ Check   ❑ Credit Card (Master Card, Visa, Amex, Discover)

Card Number:_____

Name on Card:_____ Exp. Date: ___/___

CCV Number (generally 3–4 digit number on back of card): _____

Notes

Quick Order Form

Online: http://www.SaveHerLife.com. E-book and print books—order by credit card.

Telephone orders: Call 877-432-7820 (877-HEART20) with your credit card.

Fax orders: Call 877-432-7820 to get number to fax this form.

E-mail orders: orders@saveherlife.com

Postal orders: Mellanie True Hills, Healthy Ideas Press, P.O. Box 541, Greenwood, TX 76246 Telephone: 940-466-9898

❑ Please send _____ copies of A Woman's Guide to Saving Her Own Life. I understand that I may return them for a full refund – no questions asked.

❑ Please send FREE information on Speaking/Seminars.

Name_____

Address_____

City_____ State_____ Zip_____-____

Telephone_____

E-mail address_____

Sales tax: Please add 8.25% for products shipped to Texas addresses.

Shipping:
US $5 per book
International: $10 for first book; $6 for each additional book (estimate)

Payment: ❑ Check   ❑ Credit Card (Master Card, Visa, Amex, Discover)

Card Number:_____

Name on Card:_____ Exp. Date: ___/___

CCV Number (generally 3–4 digit number on back of card): _____